Rheumatoid Arthritis Surgery of the Complex Hand and Foot

Rheumatology

An Annual Review

Vol. 11

Series Editor
M. Schattenkirchner, München

KARGER

Basel · München · Paris · London · New York · New Delhi · Singapore · Tokyo · Sydney

The 3rd Congress and General Assembly of the European Rheumatoid Arthritis Surgical Society (ERASS), Heinola, June 27–29, 1985

Rheumatoid Arthritis Surgery of the Complex Hand and Foot

Volume Editor
F.-W. Hagena, München

94 figures and 63 tables, 1987

KARGER

Basel · München · Paris · London · New York · New Delhi · Singapore · Tokyo · Sydney

Rheumatology

An Annual Review

Library of Congress Cataloging-in-Publication Data
Rheumatoid arthritis surgery of the complex hand and foot.
(Rheumatology; vol. 11)
Papers presented at the Third Congress of ERASS, held at Heinola, Finland on 27–29 June 1985.
Includes bibliographies and index.
1. Hand – Surgery – Congresses. 2. Foot – Surgery – Congresses. 3. Rheumatoid arthritis – Surgery – Congresses. I. Hagena, F.-W. (Frank W.) II. European Rheumatoid Arthritis Surgery Society. Congress (3rd: 1985: Heinola, Finland)
[DNLM: 1. Arthritis, Rheumatoid – surgery – congresses. 2. Foot – surgery – congresses. 3. Hand – surgery – congresses. W1 RH42G v. 11/WE 346 R47391 1985]
RC927.A1R5 vol. 11 [RD778] 616.7'23 s 86-27509 [616.7'22]
ISBN 3-8055-4408-1

Drug Dosage

The authors and the publisher have exerted every effort to ensure that drug selection and dosage set forth in this text are in accord with current recommendations and practice at the time of publication. However, in view of ongoing research, changes in government regulations, and the constant flow of information relating to drug therapy and drug reactions, the reader is urged to check the package insert for each drug for any change in indications and dosage and for added warnings and precautions. This is particularly important when the recommended agent is a new and/or infrequently employed drug.

Printed in Switzerland by Basler Zeitung, Basel
ISBN 3-8055-4408-1

Dedication

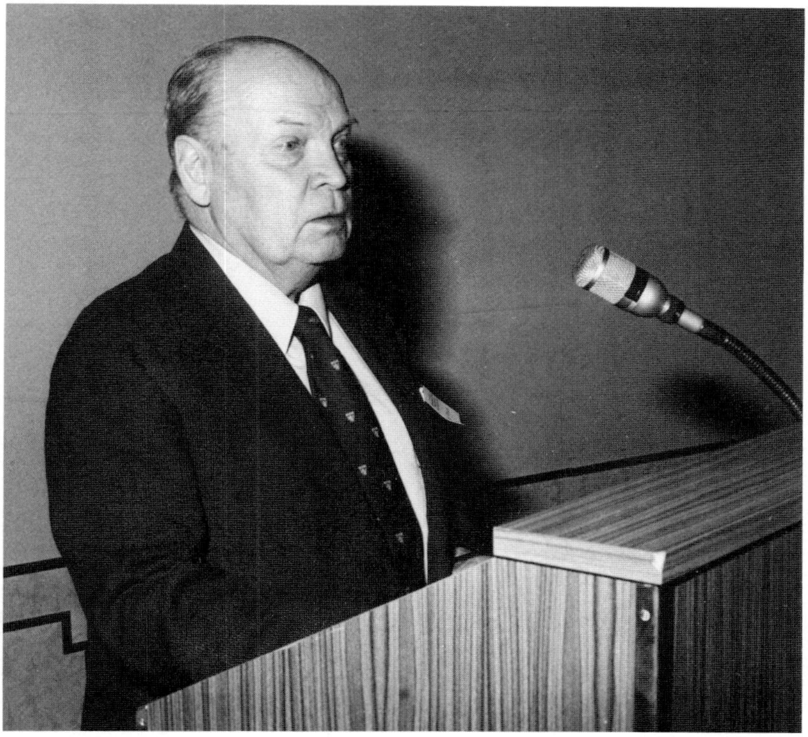

This volume is dedicated to Professor Dr. Kauko Vainio, honorary member of the European Rheumatoid Arthritis Surgical Society.

Contents

Rheumatoid Arthritis Surgery of the Complex Hand

Rheumatoid Arthritis Surgery of the Complex Foot

Preface

The age of systematic rheumatoid arthritis surgery is young, even though single procedures were performed as early as in the late 1800s. As general surgery is considered to begin in the middle of the 1800s rheumatoid arthritis surgery can be considered to begin only a hundred years later in the 1950s. Therefore rheumatoid surgery has been in a great hurry to overtake the lead of 100 years which other surgery has had. Great advances then took place during 30 odd years. Old classical orthopaedic methods were applied and new operations were created for rheumatoid arthritis.

It is of utmost importance to cooperate between the rheumatoid surgical centres in Europe and in the whole world to get significant knowledge for every surgeon performing rheumatoid operations. The material of one clinic is often too small for scientific purposes. One of the most important tasks of ERASS is just to support this collaboration. Another important task is to arrange meetings where members exchange all the news from the rheumatoid surgical field as soon as possible.

The Third Congress of ERASS was held at Heinola, Finland, on June 27–29, 1985. I am very happy that the complete papers read at the Heinola-meeting can now be published. I thank every author for preparing their paper suited for the publication. Especially I should like to thank docent F.-W. Hagena who has made every effort to get this publication ready.

Pauli Raunio
President of the 3rd ERASS Congress

Foreword

The development of joint surgery is one of the greatest advances in modern rheumatology. Within the short period of two decades, centres in different countries have designed a broad range of surgical methods with either a more preventive or a more reconstructive feature. The rapid development in this field also demands a rapid exchange of knowledge. The various method and long-term results require critical comparison. In order to make possible mutual understanding and significant evaluation, standardization is necessary.

With this objective, Professor Raunio, one of the pioneers of surgery in rheumatoid arthritis, organized the 3rd Congress of the European Rheumatoid Arthritis Surgical Society (ERASS) in Heinola in Summer 1985. The most competent experts of the world met there to present the latest achievements in 'Rheumatoid Arthritis Surgery of the Complex Hand and Foot'. The present volume contains the complete contributions of these distinguished participants.

This book certainly represents a source of up-to-date information for those rheumatologists who are engaged in rheumatic joint surgery. It is also of great assistance to the conservative rheumatologist, for therapy in rheumatology is an interdisciplinary problem. Conservative and surgical measures are inseparable parts of each therapeutic programme. Indications for the various methods of one side always depend on the possibilities of the other. This volume may be helpful in finding clear therapeutic concepts.

I am obliged to all contributors of this valuable book. My special thanks are directed to Dr. Frank-Wolfgang Hagena whose initiative, energy, and carefulness made this volume to be realized.

M. Schattenkirchner

Introduction

The Third Congress of the European Rheumatoid Arthritis Surgical Society, organized by P. Raunio, took place at Heinola, the 'Mecca' of rheumatoid arthritis surgery. International efforts on surgical treatment and especially the interdisciplinary engagement in rheumatoid arthritis are closely connected with Prof. K. Vainio, the founder of the Rheumatism Foundation Hospital in Heinola and honorary member of the ERASS, to whom this volume is dedicated.

While the Second ERASS Congress dealt with the results and possibilities of preventive surgery stressing long-term follow-up studies, the subject of the present one was to compile news and to discuss problems concerning the reconstruction of the complex function of hand and foot in RA. It is my proud honor to be able to compile up-to-date contributions from internationally known experts. I would also like to thank Prof. M. Schattenkirchner who supported and made this edition possible. It is due to friendly interdisciplinary cooperation that this important presentation could be realized. May it be an informative and helpful book for the rheumatoid and hand surgeon as well as for the rheumatologist.

Frank-W. Hagena

Rheumatoid Arthritis Surgery of the Complex Hand

Rheumatology, vol. 11, pp. 1-2 (Karger, Basel 1987)

The Complex Rheumatoid Hand: General Aspects

Lennart G. Mannerfelt

Hand-Unit, Goldenbühl Hospital, Villingen,
Affiliated University of Tübingen, FRG

Because the word *complex* is both a substantive and an adjective the word could be confusing. As a substantive it stands for a group of closely related parts, for instance buildings. We also know about Freud's and Adler's complex. Oedipus complex or inferiority complex.

As adjective it means, difficult to understand or confusing. *Complex* could also be understood as more than one problem. Finally, according to some dictionaries, *complex* stands for differentiated, complicated and intricate. Based on the definitions mentioned above, the complex rheumatoid hand is difficult to understand and confusing. The complex rheumatoid hand consists of more than one problem, it is differentiated, complicated and intricate.

What is not complex? For instance a tenosynovitis of a flexor tendon in the palm is only *one* problem, thus not complex. But, when untreated, resulting in a flexor tendon rupture, combined with metacarpophalangeal (MP) joint destructions, it could be complex in the future!

As an example of a *complex* rheumatoid hand, we can chose a patient with totally destroyed wrist joint, whereby the carpus and the hand is dislocated volarly of the distal radius and added to that all fingers are destroyed. There is no stability in the finger joints and the grip function is lost. This is the so-called 'mutilans type'. Such a patient could be helped with arthrodesis of the wrist joint and some finger joints. The patient is able to use her hand a little bit more. As Bunnell said - when you have nothing a bit is a lot.

A real complex rheumatoid hand is the late, nearly petrified hand in a case of psoriatic disease, a condition closely connected with rheumatoid arthritis. In such a patient the wrist joint is contracted in flexion position, there is no pronation at all, the tumb is valueless in adduction and hyperextension and the four ulnar fingers are 'petrified' in extension or slight recurvated in their proximal interphalangeal (PIP) joints.

To give such a patient some sort of grip function, staged procedures are necessary: in the first sitting a wrist arthrodesis combined with excision of the ulnar head to give proper pronation is required. In the second seance MP joints arthroplasty together with arthrodesis of the PIP joints in slight flexion is to be recommended.

Because of the pronounced contracted skin dorsally over the PIP joints, after the PIP arthrodesis, skin plasties with transposition - rotational flaps and reconstructions of the secondary defects with skin grafts are not seldom necessary. After having got some sort of flexion/extension function in the MP joints (arthroplasty) the thumb is reconstructed to give an abduction with proper pronation to meet the ulnar fingers when gripping. The patient now can place her hand in the desired pronated position when gripping and because her elbow joint has a ROM of 0–10–95 with an appropriate shoulder mobility she also can reach her mouth with her reconstructed hand. Combined lesions with extensor tendon ruptures and destroyed MP joints II–V require intricate surgery supported by dynamic splints (see chapter Timing in Surgery of the Rheumatoid Hand).

Lennart G. Mannerfelt, MD, Hand Unit, Goldenbühl Hospital,
D-7730 VS-Villingen (FRG)

Rheumatology, vol. 11, pp. 3–5 (Karger, Basel 1987)

Timing in Surgery of the Rheumatoid Hand

Lennart G. Mannerfelt

Hand-Unit, Goldenbühl Hospital, Villingen,
Affiliated University of Tübingen, FRG

There are different indications for surgery of the rheumatoid hand, be it: (1) preventive; (2) pain; (3) function loss; (4) cosmetic.

Nevertheless, it should always be kept in mind that surgery for so-called academic reasons (for instance destructions on the X-ray) without pain, without function loss or without claim for cosmetics seldom is indicated.

According to problems of timing, some authors, as Mr. Souter, Edinburgh, start with a 'winner'. A winner could be a dorsal synovectomy of the wrist with the excision of the ulnar head, a thumb metacarpophalangeal (MP) arthrodesis, or a carpal tunnel splitting with a flexor tenosynovectomy.

It has shown very valuable to start with a 'winner' to gain the confidence of the patient in beginning of a larger reconstruction problem. We recommend certain operations over doubtful, one should probably start with the minor hand over major, that is the nondominant hand before the dominant, when both hands are equally afflicted.

In cases of combined problems as seen in the wrist, MP and proximal interphalangeal (PIP) joints, nerves, extensors and flexors, it seems reasonable now that the wrist should be done prior to more distal surgery. It does not seem to make sense to do an arthroplasty of the MP joint or at the interphalangeal joint level in an attempt to improve motion and grip strength there – if the wrist is painful. For this reason, if all things are equal, we tend to recommend wrist surgery in an attempt to provide stability and relief of pain before operating distally.

If the patient has a button hole deformity at the PIP level, it seems reasonable that this joint should be treated prior to MP joints. The presence of a severe flexion deformity at the PIP level reduces the prognosis of MP surgery. With the PIP joints in flexion, the patients tend to keep the MP joints extended or hyperextended and do not get a good range of motion in the sense of flexion. Therefore, faced with this combination, it is sound to restore extension of the PIP joints prior to MP joint surgery.

When a patient has swan-neck deformity of Fearnly degree II or III, we feel that the MP joint gets priority in this regard. The stiffness of the PIP joint in extension is actually helpful in regaining MP joint motion. After having achieved good MP range of motion we attack the stiff PIP joint.

When the patient has combined extensor tendon ruptures as well as MP flexion contracture, luxation or destruction, it is inadequate to repair the extensor tendon rupture, if the MP joints cannot be passively extended. Faced with this combination, we tend to do the arthroplasty of the MP joints prior to the extensor tendon repairs. Following the arthroplasty of the MP joints dynamic splinting is used to substitute the missing extensors.

After having got confidence of the reconstructed MP joints the patient can actively flex and with the orthosis she can passively extend. She now becomes a good candidate for the second surgical procedure including restoration of extensor tendon function. Of course the same is true when we are talking about flexor tendon ruptures.

When dealing with thumb problems, combined with function loss of the four ulnar fingers, we believe that the four ulnar fingers should at first be reconstructed. Only thereafter, when we can see what we have gained by these ulnar operations, the thumb will be reconstructed and thereby being placed in an optimal opposing grip position towards the four ulnar fingers – most often by an arthrodesis of the MP joint in a proper pronation/rotation position.

Prof. Dr. N. Gschwend, Zürich, Switzerland, has given us a good help in the approach towards timing operations in the rheumatoid hand. When seeing a patient for the first time, he just asks the patient for her most desirable wishes. Perhaps she only complains of pain from a carpal tunnel syndrome and a thumb instability, and nothing else. In such a case let us do these two operations and neglect other deformities.

Finally, we must accept the cosmetic problems. We all know that there are women who isolate themselves from social life because of the fact that they feel that their hand looks ugly. Nevertheless, it is interesting to see how much we can gain cosmetically when we restore function of damaged parts in the body, be it in the face or in the hands. So, when reconstructing damaged rheumatoid hands we not seldom simultaneously gain cosmetically. This is also an aspect in analyzing indications for and timing of surgery.

Conclusions

Start with a 'winner'. Take the wrist prior to distal joints. Reconstruct button hole deformity prior to MP joints. Let the MP joints be reconstructed prior to extensor and flexor tendon ruptures. Make the extensor tendon or the flexor tendon reconstruction after the MP reconstruction. Let the MP work come prior to stiffened PIP joints. By difficult thumb problems, connected with deformities of the four ulnar fingers, we recommend to repair the four ulnar fingers first and thereafter place the thumb in a proper opposed grip position. Cosmetics should not be neglected but it should be recalled that cosmetics automatically gain after adequate reconstructive surgery. Each patient deserves individual consideration.

Acknowledgements

The above-mentioned statements according to 'Timing in Surgery of the Rheumatoid Hand' are stronlgy influenced from collaboration with Edward Nalebuff, Boston, USA, and through the article: Planning Treatment of the Rheumatoid Hand, The Hand, Vol. 11, No. 1, 1979, by William A. Souter, Edinburgh, UK, for which I thank these two surgeons.

Lennart G. Mannerfelt, MD, Hand Unit, Goldenbühl Hospital,
D-7730 VS-Villingen (FRG)

Rheumatology, vol. 11, pp. 6–27 (Karger, Basel 1987)

The Complex Hand

Treatment Considerations and Priorities of Finger Deformities

Alfred B. Swanson, Genevieve de Groot Swanson
Grand Rapids, Mich., USA

Multiple involvement of the interphalangeal and metacarpophalangeal joints, of the wrist, and of the tendon system by the rheumatoid disease process may result in severe and complex hand deformities. Associated disabilities of the elbow, shoulder, and of the joints of the lower extremity are frequent. These patients present with severe loss of function and are often incapable of independent activity. Restoration of function to the arthritic presents a formidable challenge; it is the responsibility of the surgeon to devise an integrated treatment program that considers the patient's possibilities for improvement and the staging of the reconstructive program.

Patient Selection and Surgical Staging

If a patient with upper and lower extremity involvement is confined to a wheelchair and has a reasonable potential for ambulation, surgery for the lower extremities is carried out first to allow full benefit of the rehabilitation program which will include the use of crutches. Excessive manual labor and awkward hand weight bearing as seen in some crutch walkers can destroy the delicate hand reconstructive procedures. Occasionally, if a patient has involvement of both hand and foot, or possibly moderate knee involvement, surgery of the upper and lower extremity can be performed simultaneously, using two surgical teams. In these cases, special platform crutches are used to reduce the stress applied to the reconstructed hand and wrist.

In cases of involvement of multiple joints of the upper extremity, the distal portions of the extremity are operated first; the hand is reconstructed before the elbow or the shoulder. Occasionally, when both upper extremities are involved, the distal portion of one extremity and the more proximal joints of the opposite extremity can be operated on at the same sitting to allow the patient to have at least one hand available for his personal activities. Several different procedures are frequently performed on one arm at the same surgical stage, depending on the tourniquet time available. The fingers, thumb, and occasionally the distal radioulnar or radiohumeral joints can be reconstructed at the same time [1–7, 11, 12, 14, 15, 17]. An operation on an extremity should not exceed 2 h; a stellate ganglion block is recommended if the tourniquet time should exceed 1.5 h. Precooling of the arm with ice packs as recommended by Tajima [18] can safely prolong the surgical time available under the tourniquet to as long as 3 h in our experience.

Surgical Staging in the Complex Hand

In the normal hand there is a fine balance between the muscle and tendon system and the architecture of the bone and joints through which they act. When the normal arch system of the hand is disturbed, the stability and equilibrium necessary for prehension are lost. In presence of multiple joint involvement in the hand, a sound knowledge of the pathogenesis of deformities is essential to recognize the cause of deformity and select the appropriate treatment method and staging (fig. 1).

The metacarpophalangeal joint is the key joint for finger function. However, because of their interdependence, all digital joints are important in functional adaptations of a disabled hand. Deformity of the proximal interphalangeal joint may adversely affect the results of metacarpophalangeal joint reconstruction. To maintain the balance at one finger joint, balance of the contiguous joints must be obtained to restore the longitudinal arch of the digit. Collapse deformities of the wrist have further negative effect on the distal balance of the hand by interfering with the normal function of the extrinsic muscles of the fingers.

The rheumatoid involvement can affect all the joints of the hand and wrist and frequently involves the thumb, radiocarpal or distal ra-

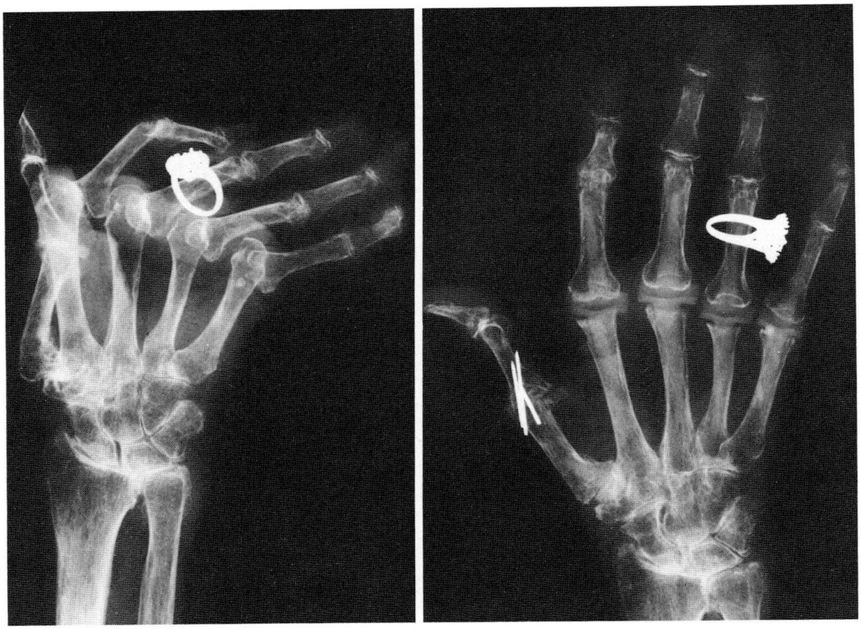

Fig. 1. a Preoperative radiogram showing a multiple finger and thumb involvement by rheumatoid arthritis and subluxation of the metacarpophalangeal joints, and swan-neck deformity of the thumb with subluxation of the carpal metacarpal joint. *b* Radiogram 2 years after implant arthroplasty of the metacarpophalangeal joints of the fingers, convex condylar implant arthroplasty at the base of the thumb, and fusion of the first metacarpophalangeal joint. The patient has a pain-free functional hand with good correction of deformities.

dioulnar joints. It is not the purpose of this presentation to detail the procedures for the wrist and thumb. Treatment of the thumb ray can require fusion or implant arthroplasty of the interphalangeal, metacarpophalangeal or basal joints of the thumb. We seldom use a trapezium implant at the basal joint level in the rheumatoid thumb; a carpal metacarpal arthroplasty with a condylar implant is preferred.

In metacarpophalangeal joint disabilities associated with severe wrist involvement, the wrist should be treated first. This may involve reconstruction of the distal radioulnar joint as well as stabilization of the carpal area either by partial fusion, semiconstrained or total wrist implant arthroplasty, or wrist fusion. Tendon repair and synovectomy of tendon sheaths should be done 6–8 weeks before joint reconstruction in the rheumatoid hand. However, if the extensor tendons are ruptured and the metacarpophalangeal joints are dislocated, arthroplasty of the metacarpophalangeal joints is done before the wrist and tendon reconstruction. In swan-neck deformity, surgery of the metacarpophalangeal and proximal interphalangeal joints are done at the same stage. However, in boutonnière deformity, it may be preferable to reconstruct the proximal interphalangeal joint before the metacarpophalangeal joint. Based on a long-term experience, a classification of treatment for combined involvement of the metacarpophalangeal and interphalangeal joints has been devised (table I) [4, 5, 17].

Metacarpophalangeal Joint

Long-standing synovitis of the metacarpophalangeal joint may result in deformation of the joint surfaces into what has been described as a 'cup-and-saucer deformity'. The base of the proximal phalanx widens and deepens centrally to receive the head of the metacarpal. The result is a relatively stable and mobile 'natural' arthroplasty, which is most frequently seen in the index and middle fingers. If these joints have adequate motion and are painfree, no further surgery is indicated. However, occasionally, resection arthroplasty may be worthwhile. Adequate bone stock must be present in the metacarpals to receive the stems of the implants. Occasionally there is inadequate bone stock to receive the finger-joint implant, especially in the little and ring fingers, due to severe bone absorption; the Tupper type of resection arthroplasty is then used for these joints. This procedure consists of detaching the palmar plate at its proximal origin, bringing it as a flap between the bone ends to the dorsal surface of the resected metacarpal shaft, and suturing it through a drill hole in the dorsal bone cortex. The collateral ligaments can also be reattached.

Metacarpophalangeal Joint Flexible Implant Arthroplasty

If implant arthroplasty is to be considered, the patient must be cooperative and in good general condition. The skin and neurovascular status must be adequate, and the elements necessary to produce a functional musculotendinous system must be available along with adequate bone stock to receive and support the implant. Adequate facilities must also be available for the operative and postoperative therapy.

Table I. Treatment of interphalangeal joint disabilities

Swan-neck deformity of PIP joint		
Without involvement of MP joint		
1. Initial deformity of PIP joint	(a) local injections (corticosteroids or other agents) (b) flexor tendon synovectomy with or without tenodesis of flexor digitorum superficialis tendon (c) intrinsic tendon release with or without flexor tendon synovectomy	
2. Flexible deformity of PIP joint	(a) dermadesis at PIP joint (b) relocation of lateral tendons with or without elongation of central tendon (c) tenodesis of flexor digitorum superficialis tendon with flexor synovectomy	
3. Rigid, subluxated or dislocated PIP joint	(a) resection of joint with relocation of lateral tendons and implant arthroplasty (rarely) (b) resection of joint and fusion	
4. Treatment for DIP joint when required in any of these conditions	(a) temporary pinning in neutral position if passively correctable (b) fusion if severely damaged or flexed	
With involvement of MP joint		
1. Flexible deformity of PIP joint	Treatment of MP Joint (a) synovectomy with proximal release of intrinsic tendons (b) relocation of subluxated joint with proximal release of intrinsic tendons (c) joint resection with proximal release of intrinsic tendons and implant arthroplasty	Treatment of PIP Joint (a) manipulation with temporary Kirschner wire fixation in flexion if required (b_1) manipulation with temporary Kirschner wire fixation in flexion if required (b_2) dermadesis (c_1) manipulation to 50° of flexion with temporary Kirschner wire fixation (c_2) relocation of lateral tendons with or without elongation of central tendon
2. Rigid, subluxated or dislocated PIP joint	Treatment of MP Joint (a) joint resection with implant arthroplasty	Treatment of PIP Joint (a) relocation of lateral tendons with elongation of central tendon (b) joint resection with fusion (c) joint resection with implant arthroplasty (rarely)
3. Treatment for DIP joint if required in any of these conditions	(a) temporary pinning in neutral position if passively correctable (b) fusion if flexion deformity is severe or articular damage exists	

Table I. (continued)

Boutonnière deformity of PIP joint			
1. Initial deformity of PIP joint		(a) local injections (corticosteroids or other agents) or splinting (b) synovectomy	
2. Flexible deformity of PIP joint		(a) reconstruction of central tendon (b) elongation of lateral tendons (c) combination of procedures a and b	with or without synovec-tomy
3. Rigid deformity of PIP joint	without bone erosion	(a joint release with reconstruction of central tendon and elongation of lateral tendons (b) joint resection with reconstruction of tendons with or without implant arthroplasty (c) distal release of lateral tendons	
	with bone erosions	(a) joint resection with reconstruction of central tendon and lateral tendons, with implant arthroplasty (b) joint resection and fusion	
4. Subluxated or dislocated PIP joint		(a) joint resection with reconstruction of central tendon and lateral tendons, with implant arthroplasty (b) joint resection and fusion	
5. Treatment of DIP joint if required in any of these conditions		(a) distal release of lateral tendons (b) fusion	

Stiff osteoarthritic PIP joint	
1. Nondislocated PIP joint	(a) joint resection with implant arthroplasty
2. Subluxated or dislocated PIP joint	(a) joint resection with implant arthroplasty (b) joint resection with fusion
3. Treatment for DIP joint if required in either of these conditions	(a) fusion if needed

Indications. Metacarpophalangeal joint implant arthroplasty is indicated in painful rheumatoid or post-traumatic disabilities presenting fixed or stiff metacarpophalangeal joints, X-ray evidence of joint destruction or subluxation, ulnar drift not correctable by soft tissue surgery alone, contracted intrinsic and extrinsic musculature and ligament system, and associated stiff interphalangeal joints [1–8, 12, 17].

Technique. A transverse skin incision is made over the metacarpal necks. The dorsal veins between the metacarpal heads are preserved. The extensor hood of the index finger is incised between the extensor digitorum communis and indicis proprius tendons; in the middle and ring fingers it is incised on the ulnar side, parallel to the extensor tendon and in the little finger, between the extensor digitorum communis and minimi tendons. The hood fibers and capsule are dissected and preserved. The metacarpal neck is exposed subperiosteally, transected with an air drill or motor saw, leaving part of the metaphyseal flare, and removed with the hypertrophied synovium. A pituitary rongeur is useful to complete the synovectomy.

A comprehensive soft tissue release procedure is done to allow the base of the proximal phalanx to be displaced above the metacarpal. The ulnar collateral ligament is released from its phalangeal insertion in all fingers; if severely contracted it can be excised with the palmar plate when necessary. At the level of all fingers the radial collateral ligament insertions are preserved whenever possible. If necessary to detach this ligament, it should be reattached to bone, as described later. The ulnar intrinsic tendon is pulled up into the wound with a blunt hook and sectioned at the myotendinous junction if tight; however, this tendon normally applies a supinatory force to the index and middle fingers and must be preserved whenever possible to avoid a postoperative pronation tendency. If indicated, the flexor sheath is incised longitudinally in its dorsal aspect and the long flexor tendon is pulled up with a blunt hook; a partial synovectomy, tendon sheath release or injection of corticosteroids can be done as needed. The abductor digiti

---

Fig. 2. a Design features of our distributing-loan flexible-hinge finger-joint implant. The distal stem is shown on the right and the proximal stem on the left. A compromise between flexibility and stiffness is achieved by proper distribution of the material at the midsection. These implants have been tested for more than 600 million flexion repetitions without evidence of fatigue failure. They are available in 11 sizes. *b* The metacarpal heads are removed, with part of the flair of the metaphysis being left. A synovectomy of the joint is performed. It is essential to completely reduce the joint by resection of bone and release of all soft-tissue contractures. *a, b* From ref. [19]. *c* On passive extension of the joint, there should be no impingement of the midsection of the implant by the bone edges. The end of the implant stems should not abut against the ends of the intramedullary canals. If necessary, the tips of the stems are shortened to allow adequate implant gliding and prevent buckling.

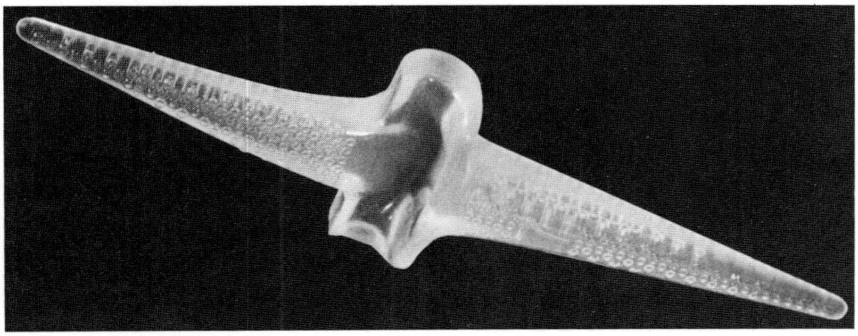

a

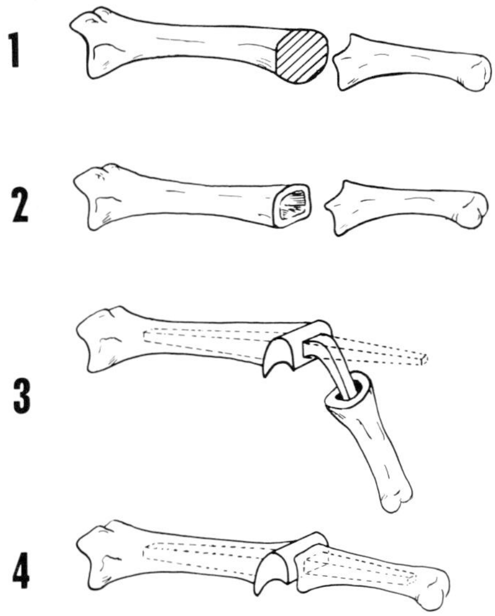
1
2
3
4

b

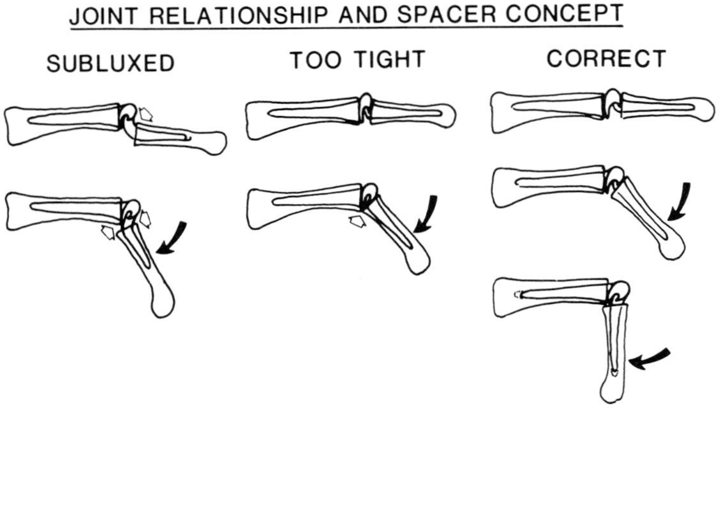
JOINT RELATIONSHIP AND SPACER CONCEPT
SUBLUXED
TOO TIGHT
CORRECT

c

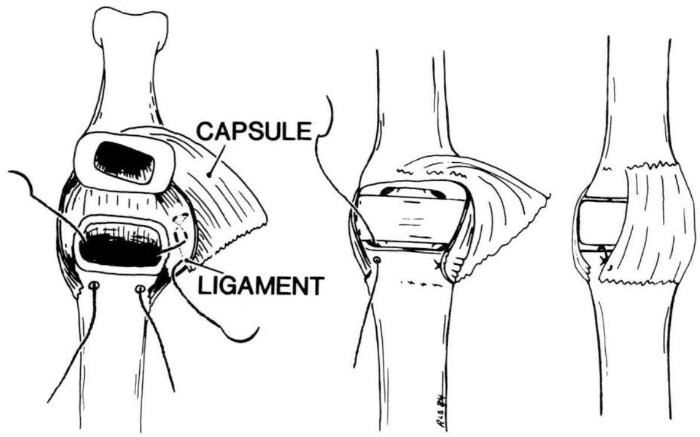

Fig. 3. Measures to correct pronation deformity of the index and middle fingers. *a* Proper rectangular and axial reaming of the intramedullary canal is necessary to stabilize the implant stems and maintain slight supination. The axis of the rectangle is placed high on the dorsal ulnar side of the base of the proximal phalanx and low on its radial palmar side. The collateral ligament and related structures are sutured to the dorsoradial aspect of the metacarpal end through a small drill hole. Sutures are placed before implant insertion. *b* Suture of radial collateral ligament. *c* Suture of the preserved radial capsule. This reconstruction further helps maintain supination of these digits.

minimi tendon is exposed on the ulnar aspect of the fifth metacarpophalangeal joint, pulled into the wound with a blunt hook, and sectioned, avoiding the ulnar digital nerve; when increased flexion power of the little finger is desired, it can be reattached through a small drill hole made in the base of the proximal phalanx. The flexor digiti minimi tendon is preserved because it is an important flexor of this joint.

The base of the proximal phalanx is resected, including marginal osteophytes or severe deformities, which might interfere with the implant. All cartilage is removed because progressive cartilage degeneration could result in recurrent synovitis. The metacarpal intramedullary canal is prepared in a rectangular fashion with a curet, broach, and air drill with a smooth leader point bur to prevent inadvertent perforation through the cortex. Too much reaming of the canal should be avoided. Using test implants, the proper size is selected so that the stem fits well into the canal and the midsection abuts against the bone end (fig. 2). The largest implant possible should be used (usually sizes 4 through 9).

The intramedullary canal of the proximal phalanx is similarly reamed. The bone must not be splintered, and any sharp points or rough surfaces should be smoothened. Proper fit of the implant is verified; with the joint in extension, there should be no impingement of its midsection. If there is, soft tissue release or bone resection has not been adequate. In the index and middle fingers the intramedullary canal of the proximal phalanx is reamed in a proper rectangular and axial configuration to stabilize the implant stems and help maintain slight supination of the digit to help prevent postoperative pronation deformity as shown in figure 3. Contrarily, in the little finger, a position of slight pronation is desired, and the intramedullary rectangle is positioned high on the dorsoradial side and low on the ulnar palmar side.

Rheumatoid patients often have an inadequate first dorsal interosseous muscle or have a tendency for pronation deformitiy of the index finger [13]. Reconstruction of the radial collateral ligament is important to correct the lateral and rotatory alignment and to improve lateral stability for pinch. The preserved radial collateral ligament of index, middle and occasionally ring finger is reattached to the metacarpal neck with a 3.0 Dacron suture passed through a 0.5-mm drill hole made on the dorsal radial side of the cut end of the metacarpal (fig. 3). This ligament can require reattachment to bone proximally (metacarpal) or distally (proximal phalanx) or to both areas according to how much bone has been removed. The preserved radial capsule is also included in this repair; it can be sutured to the dorsal ulnar side of the cut end of the metacarpal with a 4.0 Dexon suture passed through a 0.5-mm drill hole. However, it is preferred to suture the ulnar edge of the capsule to the ulnar collateral ligament to bring the repaired capsule well ulnarward over the joint. Note that the first dorsal interosseous muscle fibers become dorsally relocated with this repair. This procedure seems to decrease flexion of the metacarpophalangeal joint by 10–20 degrees by tightening the capsule, but remains important to correct pronation deformities and provide improved lateral stability for pinch. If the radial collateral ligament has been released, it should be similarly reattached. A palmar plate flap may be used to reconstruct an inadequate radial collateral ligament.

All sutures for reattachment of ligament and capsule are placed prior to implant insertion. The wound is then thoroughly irrigated, and the implant is first inserted in the intramedullary canal of the metacarpal and then into the proximal phalanx using blunt instruments and a 'no-touch' technique. With the implant in place, the sutures for radial collateral reconstruction are securely tied, inverting the knots, as the finger is held in slight supination and abduction; proper tension of the collateral ligament and radial capsule is obtained. The radial portion of the extensor hood is reefed in an overlapping fashion to bring the extensor tendon slightly to the radial side of the midline, using three to five 4-0 Dexon sutures with buried knots. In the index and middle fingers it is important not to overcorrect the extensor tendon radially to avoid creating a pronatory force. In certain cases of severe or long-standing flexion deformity, the extensor tendon should also be reefed longitudinally to correct any residual extensor tendon lag. Exceptionally, an extensor tendon tenodesis to the base of the proximal phalanx through small drill holes is indicated. The juncturae tendinae which have been divided during extensor tendon release are reapproximated with 4-0 Dexon sutures. Perfect balance of the extensor mechanism is essential.

The incision is closed and several small silicone strip drains are placed under the skin. A voluminous hand conforming dressing is applied, avoiding pressure on the radial side of the index; it includes a narrow palmar plaster splint.

Postoperative Care and Bracing. Immediate and continuous elevation of the hand and the forearm during the postoperative course is very important. On the second day the drains are usually removed. Dynamic bracing can begin on the third to fifth postoperative day (fig. 4). The rubber band slings are placed on the proximal phalanges to guide the alignment of the digits into a slight radial direction to prevent recurrent ulnar drift. The tension of the rubber band should be tight enough to support the digits and yet loose enough to allow 70 degrees of active flexion; this is especially true of the little finger, which may have weak flexion power. A thumb outrigger bar is usually applied because the patient tends to bring the thumb over the fingers on flexion and aggravate the tendency toward ulnar drift. If there is a pronation tendency of the metacarpophalangeal joint of the index finger, additional outrigger bars are applied to provide a supinatory force to the joint (fig. 4). The extension portion of the brace is worn day and night for the first 3 weeks, alternating with specific flexion exercises started 3 days after surgery. In the second week, if there is flexor weakness and good extension, the extensor sling can be removed 1–2 h a day to

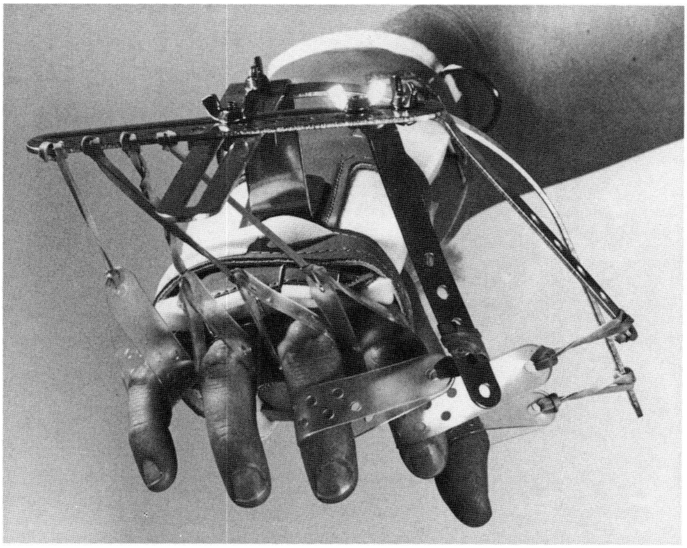

Fig. 4. Finger slings of dynamic splint are placed on proximal phalanges to assist metacarpophalangeal joint extension and guide alignment of digits. Slings are adjusted to pull from radial side to prevent ulnar deviation. Padding underneath splint with lightweight dressing or dorsal strip of felt may be necessary. Rubber bands should be loose enough to allow 70° of flexion at metacarpophalangeal joint especially of little finger. If flexion strength is weak, slings must be removed periodically to allow full range of motion. Here additional lateral slings are shown on the distal phalanx of the index and middle fingers to assist in correction of pronation deformity by forming a couple-producing supinatory torque force without interfering with flexion and extension movements. From ref. [20].

achieve greater active flexion of the metacarpophalangeal joints. In patients with normal proximal interphalangeal joints, small padded aluminum splints are taped on the dorsum of the proximal interphalangeal joints to help localize all flexion force at the metacarpophalangeal joints. At 3 weeks a flexion cuff may be worn for 1–2 h twice a day to flex the metacarpophalangeal joints passively. Other preferred traction devices used to improve flexion in the presence of adequate extension, include flexor slings applied to the proximal phalanges, or rubber bands attached from glued-on nail hooks, pulling to a special wrist

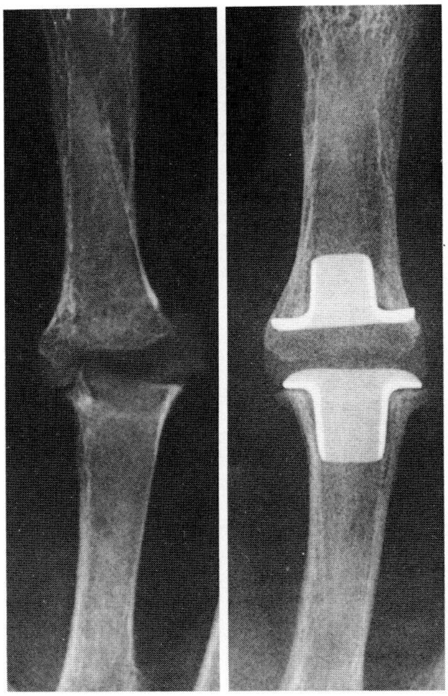

a b

Fig. 5. ***a*** Radiograph of an metacarpophalangeal arthroplasty showing the cutting effect of a sharp metacarpal bone edge into the silicone implant. ***b*** Postoperative radiogram 24 months after metacarpophalangeal implant arthroplasty using a proximal and distal grommet. Note the increased favorable bone production and remodeling around the grommet.

strap. The extension portion of the brace is usually worn at night only, starting on the fourth postoperative week for another 3 weeks or even longer as needed. A continued exercise and stretching program is followed for 3 months postoperatively. The reader is urged to refer to previous detailed publications in order to properly understand this most important rehabilitation program [9].

Grommet Bone Liners. Flexible hinge silicone implant arthroplasty has received wide acceptance as the preferred method for reconstructive surgery of the finger joints. However, implant fracture has been known to occur in approximately 5–7% of the cases [3, 7, 8, 10]. Implant tears are most often initiated by pinching or cutting of the implant by sharp bone edges across a tight subluxating joint or a joint that has become loosened through recurrent synovitis. In a joint that presents a tendency for subluxation, the implant midsection becomes impinged by the bone ends. The tendency for subluxation can be attributable to inadequate surgical correction of the deformity or to increased progression of the synovial disease; this can also be seen when the more proximal joints fall victim to the destructive process resulting in collapse of the longitudinal arch with secondary tendon imbalances distally as seen in the swan-neck deformity. In an effort to protect the implants from the cutting effect of sharp thin bone edges in certain severe rheumatoid patients, a titanium grommet was developed in our research department (fig. 5) [6].

Grommet Technique. The grommet is a press-fit bone liner contoured to fit the shape of the midsection and stems of the flexible implant. The distal grommet is placed dorsally and the proximal grommet palmarly. When using grommets, the resected surfaces of the metacarpal and proximal phalanx are shaped to obtain a precise fit of the grommet sleeve in the intramedullary canal and of its slightly curvilinear flanges against the resected bone ends. The base of the proximal phalanx is slightly grooved laterally to allow proper fit of the flanges taking care to observe the proper rotatory alignment. Fitting of the proximal grommet requires very little additional shaping of the metacarpal end. Fitting of the implant/grommet should be observed in both flexion and extension; the implant must slide under the distal grommet and not be impinged by it. The grommet is gently pushed or tapped in position with a curved instrument to avoid distorting it. If the grommet is too loose, the next larger size is used; however, a grommet smaller than the implant must never be used. If too much bone has been removed from either side of the joint, fitting of the grommet could be difficult. Careful evaluation of the radiograms before and at surgery helps determine the appropriate level of bone resection. This is particularly true in patients with severe metacarpophalangeal joint dislocation because considerable bone must be removed to realign the joint.

Grommet Contraindications. If the cut end of the metacarpal is proximal to the metaphysis, into diaphyseal bone, fitting of the grommet is difficult and the implant is inserted without a grommet. This situation can occur at the metacarpal or phalangeal level, or both.

Proximal Interphalangeal Joint

Treatment of the proximal interphalangeal joint varies with the type and severity of deformity presented and associated deformities of contiguous joints as listed in table I. The joint can be stiff without collapse deformity, with or without lateral deviation or there can be either a swan-neck or a boutonnière deformity.

Patients with synovial hypertrophy of the proximal interphalangeal joint, associated with a mild or moderate boutonnière or swan-neck deformity in which there is no radiographic evidence of erosive disease, may be candidates for soft tissue reconstructive procedures providing there is only a minimal degree of associated joint contracture. However, if subluxation, severe contracture or erosive disease of the joint is present, implant resection arthroplasty with reconstruction of the tendon mechanism or arthrodesis should be considered. It should be noted that implant arthroplasty of the proximal interphalangeal joint is never performed in presence of swan-neck deformity and only rarely done for a boutonnière deformity in the rheumatoid patient.

Soft Tissue Release Procedures

In presence of intact joint surfaces and providing joint subluxation and contracture is not too severe, the deformities can be corrected by joint release including the collateral ligament and palmar plate, joint synovectomy and repair of the extensor mechanism. In swan-neck deformity the central tendon is relatively tight and the lateral bands are displaced dorsally; in boutonnière deformity the central tendon is relatively loose and the lateral bands are displaced palmarly. Proper balance of the central tendon and lateral bands must be obtained.

Swan-Neck Deformity

In swan-neck deformity, flexor synovitis is treated prior to joint reconstruction. If the joint surfaces are preserved soft tissue release of the joint, relocation of the lateral bands palmarly, and checkrein procedures are useful to correct the deformity. In case of moderate swan-neck deformity, Zancolli and Littler's checkrein procedures are useful. In flexible hyperextension deformity of the proximal interphalangeal joint without involvement of metacarpophalangeal joint, teno-

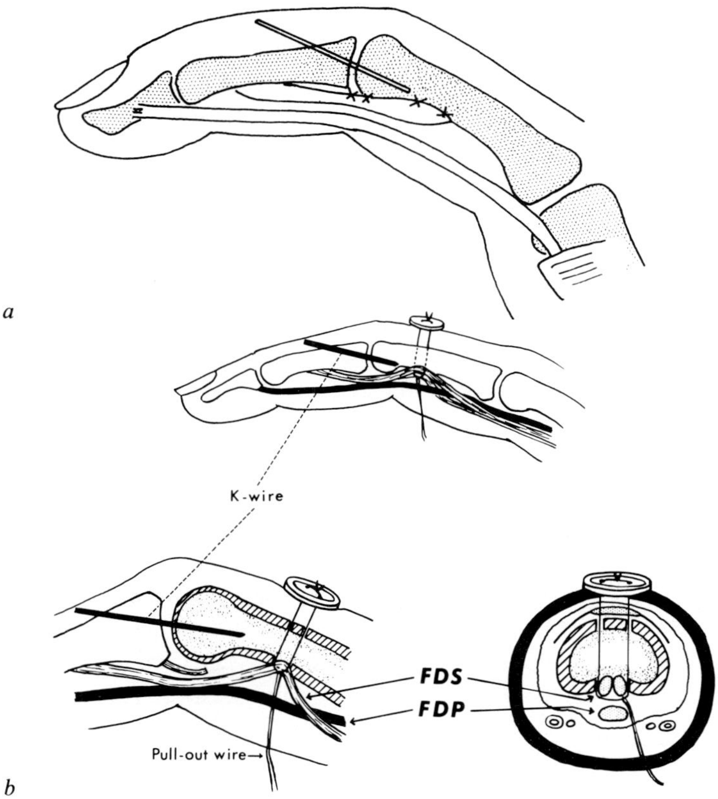

Fig. 6. Methods used in tenodesis of the flexor digitorum sublimis tendon to the proximal phalanx. In tenodesis procedures it is best to attach the tendon directly into bone. A Kirschner wire should be used to temporarily fix the proximal interphalangeal joint at the desired angle of flexion. *a* If the sublimis tendon must be resected, the stump of the tendon is used for the tenodesis. *b* If the sublimis tendon is retained, it can be tenodesed to the proximal phalanx just proximal to the bifurcation for the flexor digitorum sublimis tendon. FDS = Flexor digitorum sublimis; FDP = flexor digitorum profundus. From ref. [4].

desis of the flexor digitorum sublimis as originally described by the senior author is indicated and can be carried out at the same time as a flexor synovectomy. In mild flexible hyperextension deformity in weak hands dermadesis of the proximal interphalangeal as originally described by the senior author is indicated. In presence of combined involvement at the metacarpophalangeal and proximal interphalangeal joints, both joints are repaired at the same surgical stage. In severe cases of swan-neck deformity, joint fusion is preferred.

Flexion deformities of the distal interphalangeal must be corrected at the same time to obtain proper balance of the digit. This can be done by temporary pinning in neutral position if the deformity is passively correctable or by fusion if the joint is severely damaged.

Flexor Digitorum sublimis tenodesis. In tenodesis procedures, it is important to attach the tendon directly into bone to avoid recurrences of deformity. If the sublimis tendon is resected, the stump of the tendon is used for the tenodesis (fig. 6a). If the sublimis tendon is retained, it is tenodesed to the proximal phalanx just proximal to the bifurcation of the flexor digitorum sublimis tendon (fig. 6b). The flexor sheath is exposed at the proximal interphalangeal joint and incised longitudinally to expose the flexor tendons. The palmar plate is partially resected at its proximal portion so that it will not interfere with the tenodesis. Two small drill holes are placed approximately 0.25 inch through the palmar aspect of the neck of the proximal phalanx and connected with a currette to prepare a broad bed for attachment of the sublimis tendon. The end of the sublimis tendon is scarified and drawn up into the bone with a Bunnell type pullout suture. The tension of the tenodesis should be adjusted as to allow 20° to 30° of extension lag at the proximal interphalangeal joint. A small Kirschner wire is inserted across the proximal interphalangeal joint to maintain the desired degree of flexion throughout the healing period. The end of the wire is cut immediately under the skin, or cut so that 1 cm of wire extrudes from the skin. The cut end of the wire is capped with a plastic cap. The pullout wire is removed in 4–5 weeks and the Kirschner wire in 6–8 weeks. Small aluminum splints may be taped on the fingers to hold the proximal interphalangeal joint in flexion if the Kirschner wire needs to be removed prematurely or if further immobilization is desired.

Dermadesis. An elliptical wedge of skin can be removed from the flexor aspect of the proximal interphalangeal joint to correct a flexible hyperextension deformity in weak hands (fig. 7). Enough skin should be removed to obtain approximately 20° of flexion contracture. Great care should be taken to avoid injury to the underlying vessels and nerves.

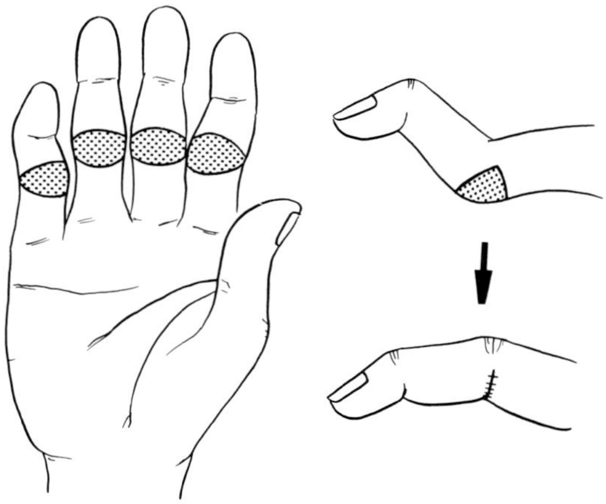

Fig. 7. The dermadesis procedure for correction of a mild flexible hyperextension deformity in weak hands. An elliptical wedge of skin is excised from the flexor aspect of the proximal interphalangeal joint, taking care to avoid the underlying nerves and vessels. Enough skin should be removed to create a flexion contracture of approximately 20°. From ref. [4].

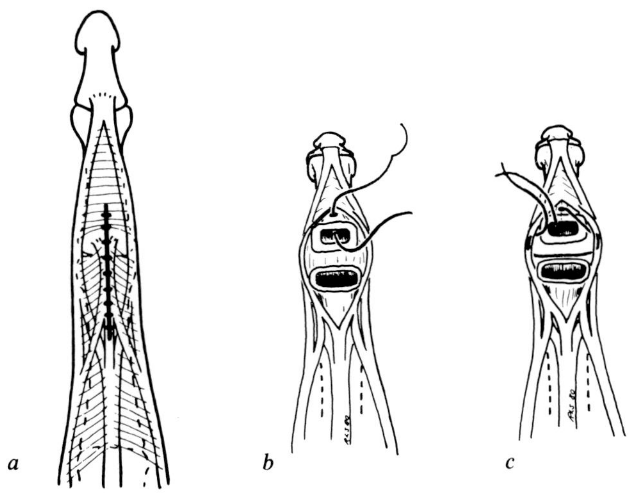

Fig. 8. Extensor tendon reconstruction. *a* Central tendon is incised longitudinally from base of proximal phalanx through distal two thirds of proximal phalanx. *b, c* Following adequate bone preparation, a 1-mm drill hole is made in base of middle phalanx to receive a 3–0 Dacron suture for reinsertion of the halves of the central tendon. In boutonnière deformity the lateral tendons are reefed dorsally using 5-0 Dexon sutures inverting the knots. From ref. [21].

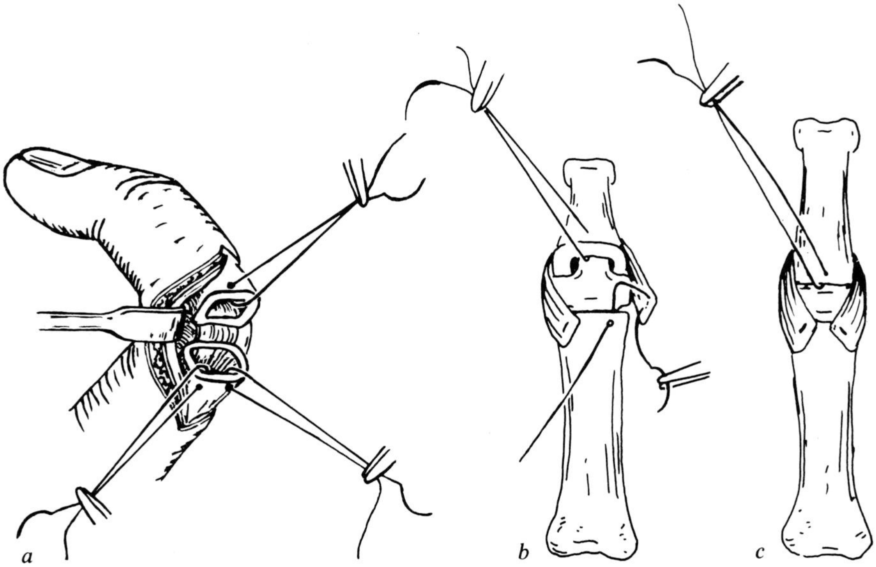

Fig. 9. Collateral ligament reconstruction. *a* 4-0 Dacron sutures are placed in the dorsal lateral aspect of the neck of the proximal phalanx for reconstruction of the collateral ligament. A 3-0 Dacron suture is placed through the base of the middle phalanx for reconstruction of the central tendon. In implant arthroplasty, sutures are placed before implant insertion. *b, c* Reattachment of the collateral ligaments. From ref. [11].

It is important in any reconstruction for swan-neck deformity to obtain a permanent flexion contracture of at least 10°. For approximately 10 days the proximal interphalangeal joint is held in about 20° of flexion with a small, taped-on aluminum splint. Active movements are then begun and encouraged, and flexion exercises are performed while the proximal interphalangeal joint is supported. Hyperextension of the reconstructed joints must be avoided in the first 3–6 weeks so that a slight flexion contracture will develop and correction of the hyperextension deformity will be maintained.

Boutonnière Deformity

In combined involvement of the metacarpophalangeal and proximal interphalangeal joint the boutonnière deformity is preferably repaired prior to reconstruction of the metacarpophalangeal joint. If the proximal interphalangeal joint surfaces are preserved and the contrac-

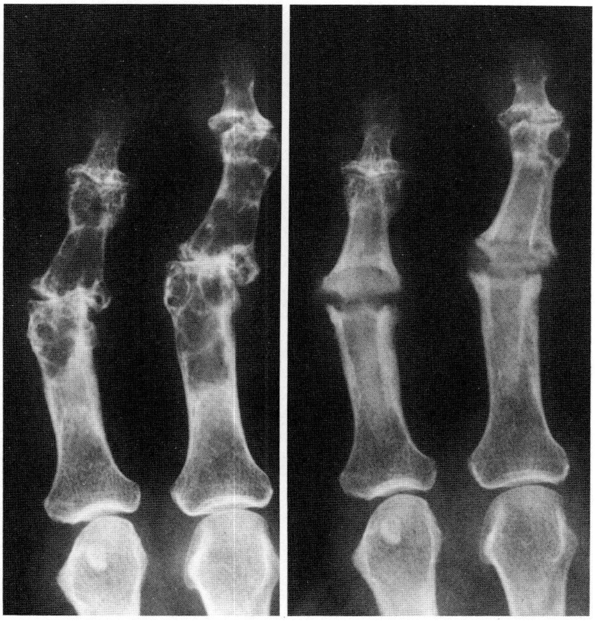

a *b*

Fig. 10. a Preoperative roentgenogram of a 72-year-old woman with painful, erosive osteoarthritis and severe cystic degenerative changes. *b* One year after surgery, the patient had a pain-free, functional arthroplasty; excellent bone healing has occurred around the implant. From ref. [11].

ture is not too severe, joint release and synovectomy, reconstruction of the central tendon and dorsal relocation of the lateral bands are indicated. If the joint surfaces are destroyed or there is severe contracture, implant arthroplasty with reconstruction of the extensor mechanism can be occasionally considered; joint fusion is, however, preferred. Correction of the hyperextension deformity of the distal interphalangeal joint must be obtained. If the distal joint cannot be flexed passively, the lateral tendons are released proximal to the insertion of Landsmeer's ligament. If the joint surfaces are destroyed, the distal interphalangeal joint is fused.

In boutonnière deformity reconstruction, repair of the extensor mechanism and the collateral ligament system is similar whether a flexible implant is used or not. The attachment of the central tendon is sutured with a 4-0 Dacron suture passed through a 0.5-mm drill hole in the base of the middle phalanx (fig. 8). The lateral tendons are released and relocated dorsally by suturing their connecting fibers or overlapping the fibers if redundant. The collateral ligaments are left intact whenever possible; if incised, they are reattached to bone (fig. 9).

The proximal interphalangeal joint is splinted in extension for 3–6 weeks. The distal joint should be allowed to flex freely. Active flexion-extension exercises are started 10–14 days after surgery in alternation with extension splinting at night which should be continued until the joint is stable; this may require 10 weeks (fig. 10).

Summary

Reconstruction of the multiple involved complex hand in the arthritic patient presents a true surgical challenge. Careful planning and staging of the surgical procedures is essential to attain adequate results.

References

1 Swanson, A.B.: Silicone rubber implants for replacement of arthritic or destroyed joints in the hand. Surg. Clins N. Am. *48:* 1113–1127 (1968).

2 Swanson, A.B.: Finger joint replacement by silicone rubber implants and the concept of implant fixation by encapsulation. Ann. rheum. Dis. *28:* suppl., pp. 47–55 (1969).

3 Swanson, A.B.: Flexible implant arthroplasty of arthritic finger joints: rationale, technique and results of treatment. J. Bone Jt Surg. *54A:* 435–455 (1972).

4 Swanson, A.B.: Flexible implant resection arthroplasty in the hand and extremities (Mosby, St. Louis 1973).

5 Swanson, A.B.: Reconstructive surgery in the arthritic hand and foot. Ciba clin. Symp. *31* (1979).

6 Swanson, A.B.: A grommet bone liner for flexible implant arthroplasty. Bull. Prosthet. Res. Rehab. Eng. Res. Devel. *1:* 108–114 (1981).

7 Swanson, A.B.; Swanson, G. de Groot: Joint replacement in the rheumatoid metacarpophalangeal joint; in Inglis, AAOS Symp. on Total Joint Replacement of the Upper Extremity, pp. 217–237 (Mosby, St. Louis 1982).

8 Swanson, A.B.; Swanson, G. de Groot; Frisch, E.E.: Flexible (silicone) implant arthroplasty in the small joints of extremities; concepts, physical and biological considerations, experimental and clinical results; in Rubin, Biomaterials in reconstructive surgery, pp. 595–623 (Mosby, St. Louis 1983).

9 Swanson, A.B.; Swanson, G. de Groot; Leonard, J.: Postoperative rehabilitation program in flexible implant arthroplasty of the digits; in Hunter, Schneider, Mackin, Bell, Rehabilitation of the hand; 2nd ed., pp. 665–680 (Mosby, St. Louis 1984).

10 Swanson, A.B.; Swanson, G. de Groot; Poitevin, L.A.; Kearney, J.: Bone remodeling phenomena in flexible (silicone) implant arthroplasty in the hand – long-term study. Kappa Delta Award Lecture. 49th Annu. Meet. of Orthopaedic Surgeons, New Orleans 1982. Orthop. Rev. *11:* 129–131 (1982).

11 Swanson, A.B.; Maupin, B.K.; Gajjar, N.V.; Swanson, G. de Groot: Long-term review of flexible implant arthroplasty in the proximal interphalangeal joint of the hand. J. Hand Surg. *10A:* 796–805 (1985).

12 Swanson, A.B.; Swanson, G. de Groot: Flexible implant arthroplasty in the rheumatoid metacarpophalangeal joint. Clin. rheum. Dis. *10:* 609–629 (1984).

13 Swanson, A.B.; Swanson, G. de Groot; Winfield, D.L.: The pronated index finger deformity in the rheumatoid hand. Bull. Hosp. Jt Dis. *44:* 498–510 (1984).

14 Swanson, A.B.; Swanson, G. de Groot: Arthroplasty of the thumb basal joints. Clin. Orthop. *195:* 151–160 (1985).

15 Swanson, A.B.; Swanson, G. de Groot; Maupin, B.K.: Flexible implant arthroplasty of the radiocarpal joint. Surgical technique and long-term study. Clin. Orthop. *187:* 94–106 (1984).

16 Swanson, A.B.; Swanson, G. de Groot: Osteoarthritis in the hand. Clin. rheum. Dis. *11:* 393–420 (1985).

17 Swanson, A.B.; Swanson, G. de Groot: Flexible implant resection arthroplasty for the rheumatoid hand and wrist. Chir. Gyn. *74:* suppl. 198, pp. 54–69 (1985).

18 Tajima, T.: Considerations on the use of the tourniquet in surgery of the hand. J. Hand Surg. *8:* 799 (1983).

19 Inglis, A. (ed.): Joint replacement in the rheumatoid metacarpophalangeal joint. AAOS Symp. on Total Joint Replacement of the Upper Extremity, pp. 217–237 (Mosby, St. Louis 1982).

20 Hunter, J.M.; Schneider, L.H.; Macklin, E.J.; Bell, J.A. (eds.): Postoperative rehabilitation program in flexible implant arthroplasty of the digits. Rehabilitation of the hand; 2nd ed., pp. 665–680 (Mosby, St. Louis 1984).

21 Swanson, A.B.: Arthroplasty in the rheumatoid hand; in Lamb, Kuczynski, Practice of hand surgery (Blackwell, Oxford 1981).

Alfred B. Swanson, MD, Blodgett Professional Building, Suite 290,
1900 Wealthy Street, SE, Grand Rapids, MI 49506 (USA)

Rheumatology, vol. 11, pp. 28–38 (Karger, Basel 1987)

Possibilities of Combining Various Operative Procedures in the Complex Hand

F.-W. Hagena, W. Bracker

Staatliche Orthopädische Klinik der Ludwig-Maximilian-Universität, München, FRG

Introduction

The drawings of Kapandji [1984] show excerpts of the amazing, complex function of the healthy hand (fig. 1). Especially in cases of so-called 'forgotten rheumatoid hands' it is impossible to restitute this function. To treat complex hand deformities the knowledge of normal patterns of the hand is as important as the understanding of the chain of the upper extremity: the cervical spine, the shoulder, the elbow and of course the wrist!

In many cases physicians are hesitant to start with operative therapy because of possible complications. So patients with rheumatoid arthritis (RA) are observed while function deteriorates extremely. Flatt [1983] showed that there is no justification for a policy of 'wait and see', if signs of early deterioration of function are recognized. Patients are able to adapt to their diminution of function over a long period. They learn tricks to help themselves as far as possible, sometimes even with very poor aids (fig. 2).

Indications

How does one set up indications for reconstructive surgery in those 'forgotten rheumatoid hands'? Because of extreme destruction of the joints, the hand and wrist dislocation is fixed; passive and active range of motion is limited. Increasing muscle atrophy enlarges instabil-

1
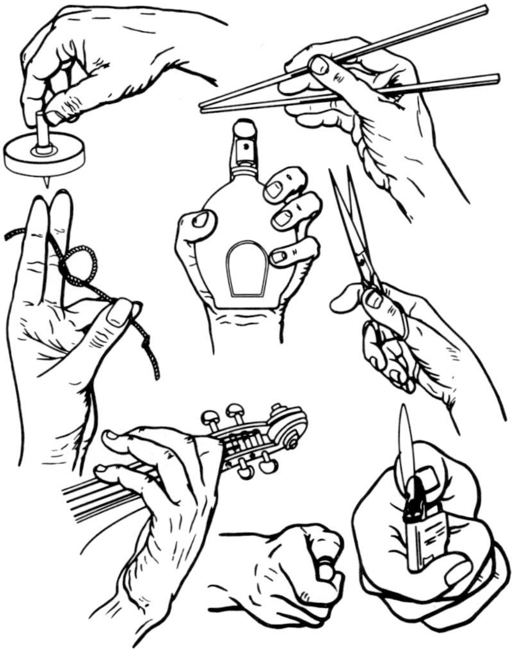

2
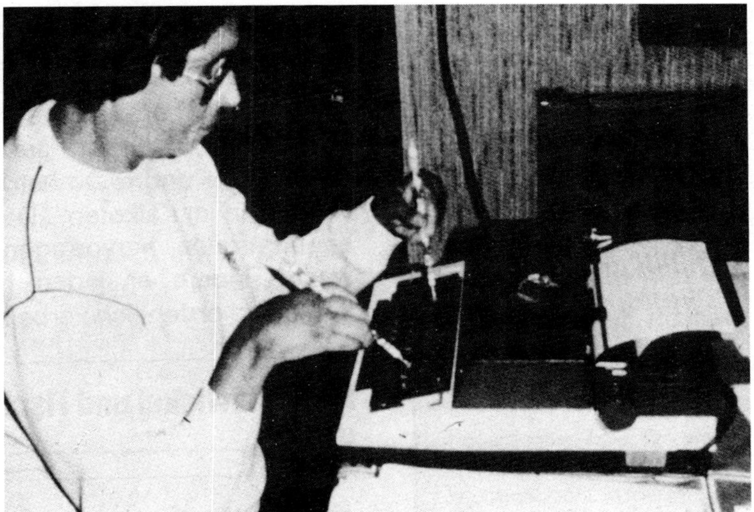

Fig. 1. Drawings adapted from Kapandji [1984].
Fig. 2. Simple sticks as aids for typewriting.

Table I. Indication for reconstructive procedures

Pain	instability
Destruction	loss of function
Dislocation	(cosmetics?)
Deficit of rom	

ity of the wrist and finger joints. In these cases we often find additional tendon ruptures. They have to be differentiated from luxations of the tendons between the metacarpophalangeal (MCP) heads. Besides pain the loss of function should be the main parameter for indicating reconstructive surgery. Sometimes patients seem to think about cosmetic aspects (table I). For example the case of a 72-year-old, strong-minded patient is shown. He was unable to help himself. The X-rays show the luxation of the wrist and MCP joints with instability of the thumb and proximal interphalangeal (PIP) joints. This is a combination of all possible and important indicating factors for reconstructive surgery of the complex hand deformity (fig. 3a, b).

First we have to question the motivation of the patient. Is he willing to undergo the reconstructive procedure and the following programme of physiotherapy and occupational therapy for a long time? Secondly, the necessarily motivated doctors who, really wanting to help their patients, should be able to stimulate the patients and aiding personal. What are the limiting factors? The indication is limited, especially by reduced vitality, class of function and when postoperative cooperation is uncertain (table II). In conclusion, with Flatt [1983] it is pointless to try to 'sell' a patient an operation! There are extremely important questions about necessity, possibility and the reason of combined procedures (table III).

Operative Procedures

Planning reconstructive surgery with a combination of different procedures in the rheumatoid hand, we need to closely examine the involvement of nerves, tendons and joints. A neurological investigation may be helpful. In cases where there are signs of lesions caused by compression of the n. ulnaris or medianus, it is a one-step procedure to

a 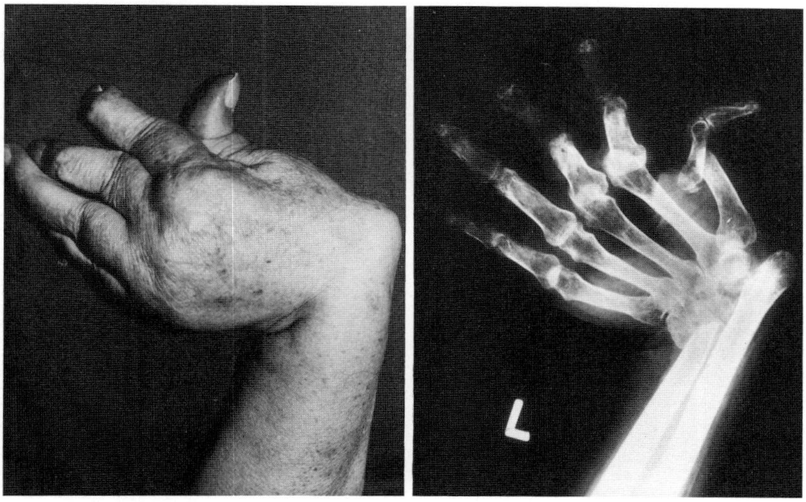 b

Fig. 3.a, b See text.

Table II. Limiting risks for operations in rheumatoid arthritis

Reduced
- Situation of vitality
- Postop. cooperation
- Class of function (ARA)

Table III. Limiting factors for reconstructive operations in rheumatoid hands

Reduced innervation	muscle atrophy/imbalance
Tendon-contracture	loss of bone

combine decompression of the nerves with tenosynovectomy of the palmar hand, first. The next step would be to look at the extensor mechanism and wrist and/or finger joints and tendons.

Transfer or suture of tendons may be combined with stabilization as an arthrodesis of the wrist and smaller finger joints. Combining several procedures we do not favour resection arthroplasty, but alloarthroplasty. Whereas resection arthroplasty may give more motion we

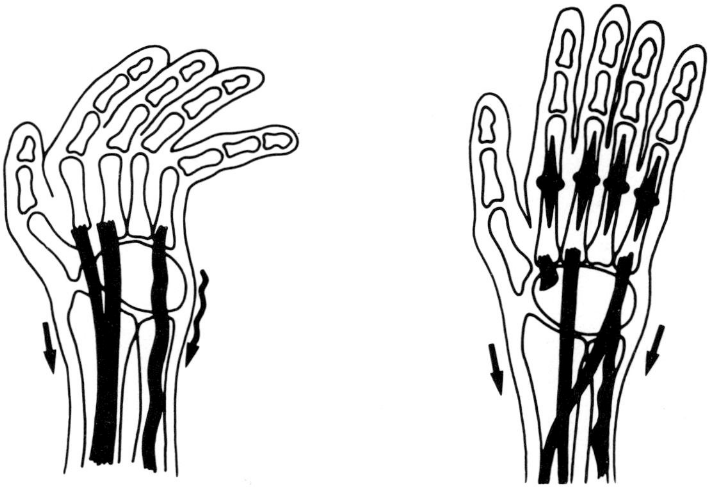

Fig. 4. Transfer of the tendons of the extensor carpi radialis to the ECU [Allieu and Brahin, 1985].

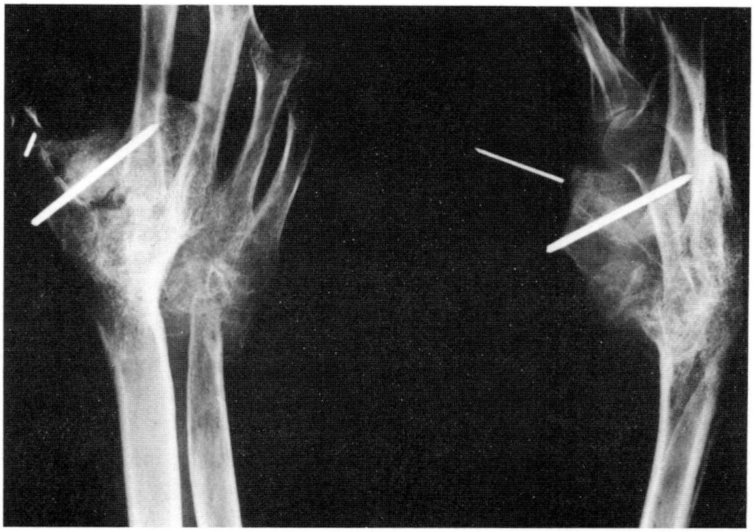

Fig. 5. See text.

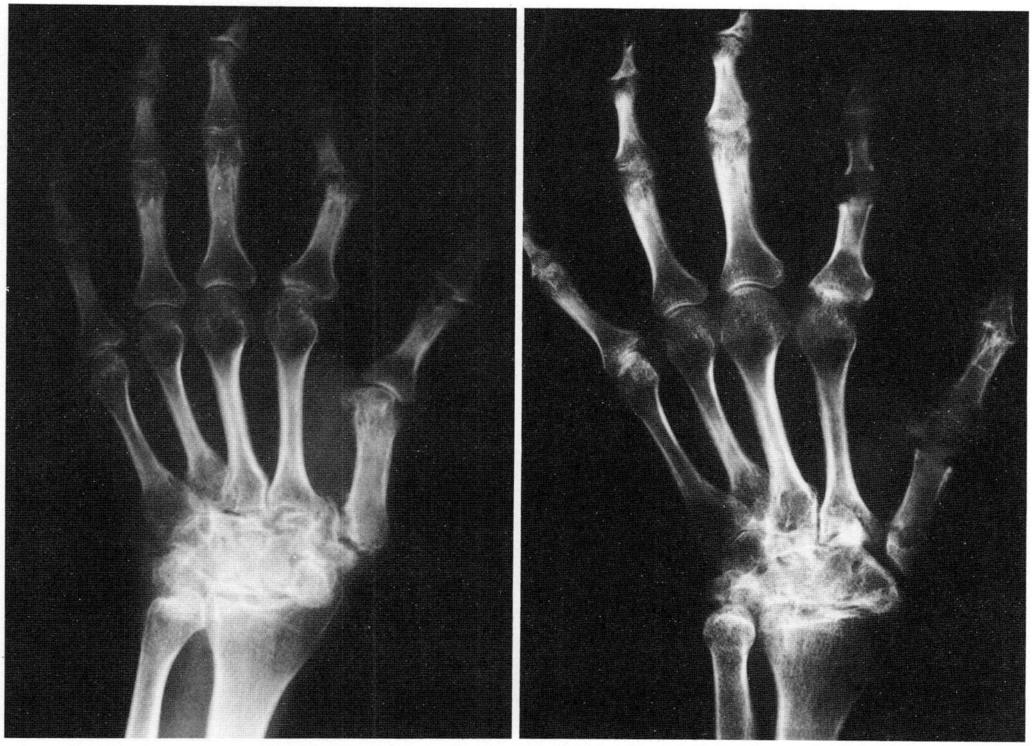

a *b*

Fig. 6. a, b See text.

think that alloarthroplasty is better because of its stability. For arthrodesis of the wrist in RA we prefer the Mànnerfelt procedure to the AO method. In some cases without detoriation of the wrist joint the transfer of the tendon of the extensor carpi radialis to the ulnar side may be helpful to correct the radial rotation of the wrist (fig. 4).

The thumb is the most important pillar for the differentiated functions of the hand. Depending on destruction of the carpal metacarpal (CMC), MCP and/or of the interphalangeal (IP) joint, we will stabilize with different kinds of operative procedures. The reconstruction of the thumb has to be planned carefully. In case of an intact CMC joint usually an arthrodesis of the MCP and IP joint gives the best result in terms of function and stability. If however there is a destruction of the CMC joint and the MCP joint, we could combine either an arthrodesis

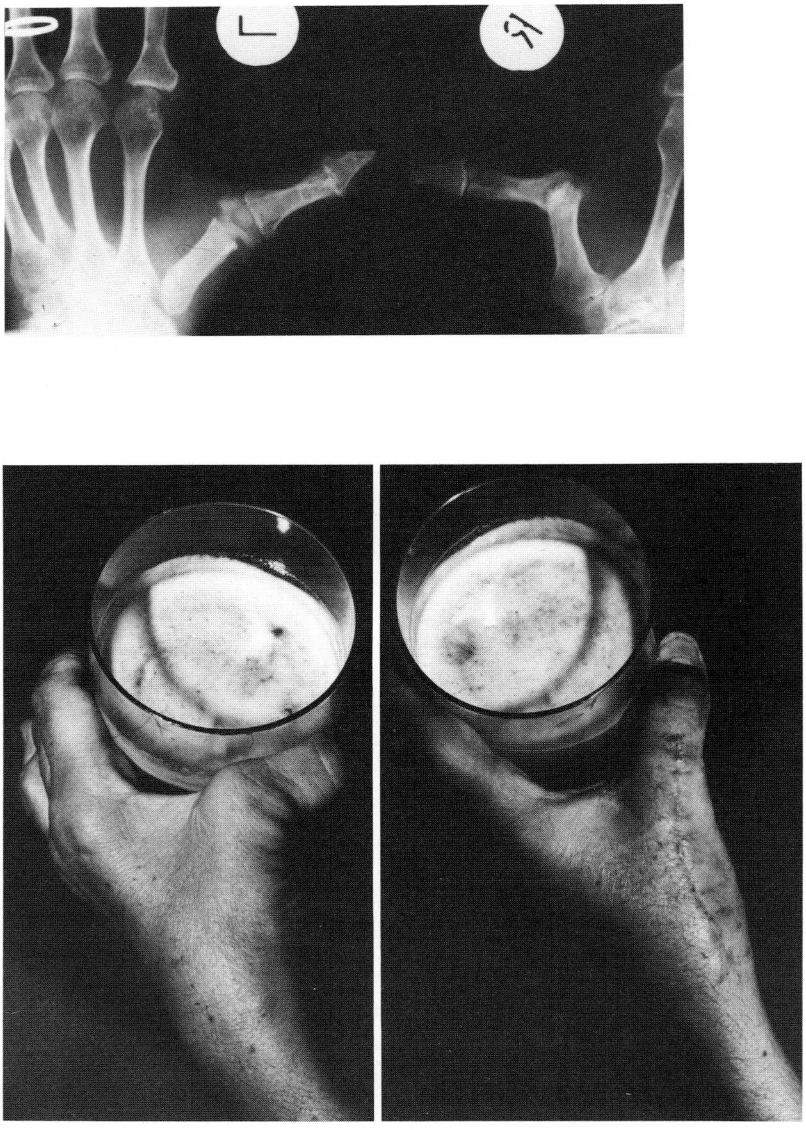

a b c

Fig. 7. Postoperative functional assessment. *a* X-Rays with abduction stress in comparison of both thumbs. *b* Clinical test holding a glass in comparison preoperative and *c* postoperative situation.

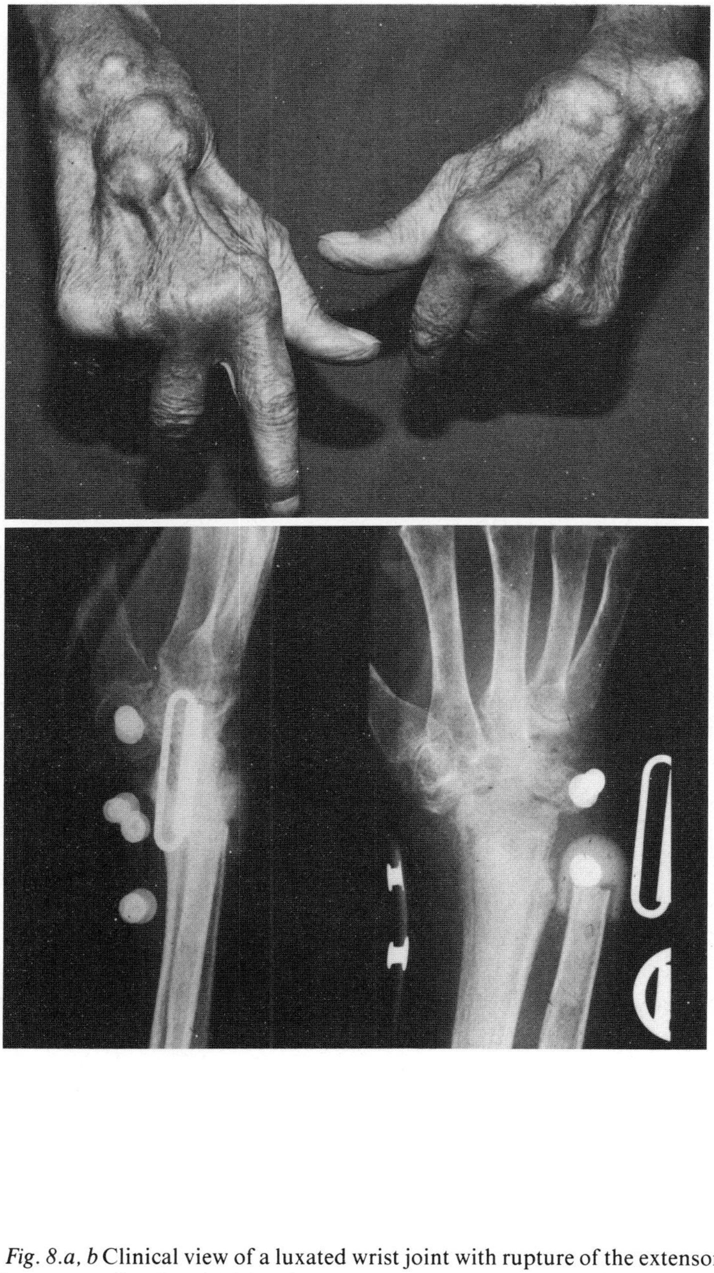

a

b

Fig. 8.a, b Clinical view of a luxated wrist joint with rupture of the extensor tendons III–V postoperative X-ray with wrist replacement by Swanson spacer and suture of the extensor tendons fixed in a splint.

of the MCP and arthroplasty of the CMC or an arthroplasty of the MCP and resection arthroplasty of the CMC. After arthrodesis of the wrist joint the intercarpal arthrodesis of os metacarpal I–III may be helpful (fig. 5).

As is demonstrated in a case of a 27-year-old typist there are extreme destructions and instability of all three joints of the thumb. In this case we replaced the MCP joint with a silastic spacer. At the distal IP joint there is no indication for a flexible hinge, but for arthrodesis. In this case there is a possibility for combining the procedure with resection arthroplasty of the MCP joint. One half of the tendon of the flexor carpi radialis is fixed at the base of metacarpal bone I to improve the mobility and the stability of the thumb (fig. 6, 7).

The combination of alloarthroplasties at the MCP and the PIP joints of the fingers is a very rare procedure. Only a fixed extension contracture of the MCP joint seems to be a possible indication for the replacement of the PIP joint.

On the other hand, there is the problem of combination of tendon sutures with different procedures at the wrist and finger joints. In general a suture of ruptured extensor tendons should be combined with arthrodesis of the wrist; in one case we did a suture of three extensor tendons and at the same time implanted a silastic wrist spacer. After so stabilizing the wrist, in a second operation the reconstruction of the MCP and PIP joints should be performed (fig. 8a, b). Especially in cases of long-lasting instability of the joints including extreme muscular atrophy it is necessary to stabilize the wrist and finger joints with arthrodesis. The MCP II–V joints and the CMC I joint are preserved for movement by implanting flexible hinges.

Showing a combination of various operative procedures in the complex hand we demonstrate the reconstruction of a luxated wrist joint and finger joints with rupture of two extensor tendons. In a two-step procedure we first could stabilize the wrist joint after resection of the base of the radius with suture of the extensor tendons. As a second step we performed Swanson replacements at the MCP II–V and an arthrodesis of MCP I, IP I, PIP II and III.

The postoperative care took about 3 months at the hospital to improve function. Three years after this operation the now 76-year-old patients is happy; he does not want to miss his left hand (fig. 9a, b).

We have to keep in mind what is possible and reasonable as a one-step procedure, depending on the palmar or dorsal side, limited by

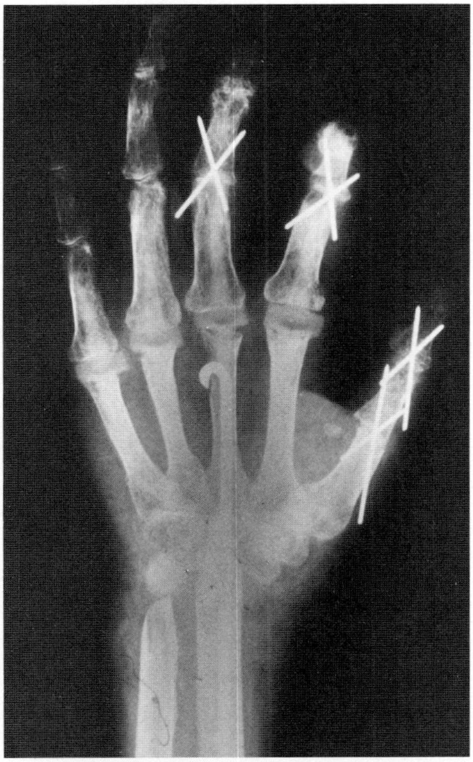

a

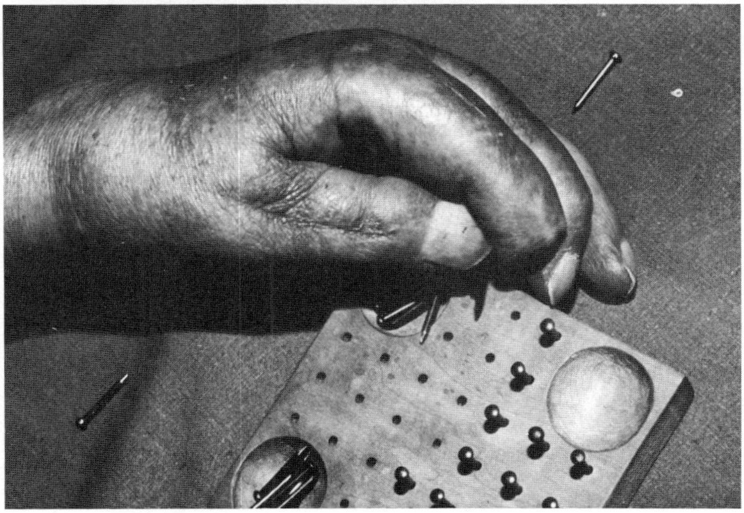

b

Fig. 9. a, b Patient 1 (fig. 3): postoperative X-ray and functional assessment.

Table IV. The combination of different steps at *one* procedure

The combination depends on
Palmar/dorsal side
Duration of operation
Possibility of postoperative care
Mobilization
Immobilization
Only one hand

risks of blood supply and the duration of operation. It is self-evident that we only operate on one hand and have to plan what we are able to do (table IV).

The coordination of tendons and muscles is very weak when there is a long enduring inactivity in a 'forgotten rheumatoid hand'. So the facilities of postoperative care and treatment have to be included in planning the reconstructive surgery.

Summary

In a complex hand deformity the combination of possible operative procedures and steps to reconstruct function depend on the chain of the upper extremity and the local conditions. The operative possibilities are limited by different factors concerning postoperative care, the patient's motivation and the doctor's experience. An exact planning of the operative procedures is a basic requirement. The combination of various procedures is discussed.

References

Allieu, Y.; Brahin, B.: Les déformations de la main rhumatoïde et leurs traitements. Documenta Geigy (1985).

Flatt, A.E.: Care of the arthritic hand; 4th ed. (Mosby, St Louis 1983).

Kapandji, I.A.: Funktionelle Anatomie der Gelenke, Bd. 1 (Bücherei des Orthopäden, Bd. 40, 1984).

Kirst, E.: Im Wohnmobil nach Dänemark. Mobil *2:* 55 (1985).

Priv. Doz. Dr. F.-W. Hagena, Rheuma-Einheit der
Ludwig-Maximilian-Universität, Staatliche Orthopädische Klinik,
Harlachingerstr. 51, D-8000 München 90 (FRG)

Rheumatology, vol. 11, pp. 39–48 (Karger, Basel 1987)

Midterm Results of the Dorsal Tenosynovectomy Including Combination Surgery of the Wrist

H.J. Refior, R. Hoos

Orthopädische Klinik der Medizinischen Hochschule Hannover, Hannover, FRG

Several investigators were able to show in as many as one third of their cases a dorsal tenosynovitis in the area of the wrist in rheumatoid arthritis [1 (Mansat, Gschwend etc.)]. Clinically this local tenosynovitis presents with pain and a hourglass like swelling. This swelling causes a pad at the distal border of the extensor retinaculum when the long fingers are extended (fig. 1). On the other hand a synovitis of the wrist leads to a homogeneous swelling up [6, 7].

By the invasive process of the inflammatorily altered tenosynovia, the affected dorsal tendons become destroyed. This is the main cause for a spontaneous rupture of the tendons in rheumatoid arthritis. Apart from that the additional mechanical stress on the dorsal side of the wrist, as on the tuberculum listeri, the luxated head of the ulna, as well as on the dorsal border of the radius (in the case of the volar luxated wrist) also has an important influence.

Because of that pathomorphology of the dorsal tenosynovitis of the wrist, all the other joints of the hand are affected, as each disturbance of the muscle balance necessarily leads to deviation and deformation [1]. Baeckdahl [1] was able to show by means of pathologic-anatomical, arthrographical and electromyographical investigations that the extensor carpi ulnaris muscle is the only extensor of the hand which stabilises the distal radial-ulnar joint even in the case of volar flexion. This function, however, is lost if it is affected by chronic tenosynovitis as well, thus resulting in a caput-ulna syndrome. We see this condition fairly frequently since an isolated tenosynovitis occurs very often in rheumatoid arthritis.

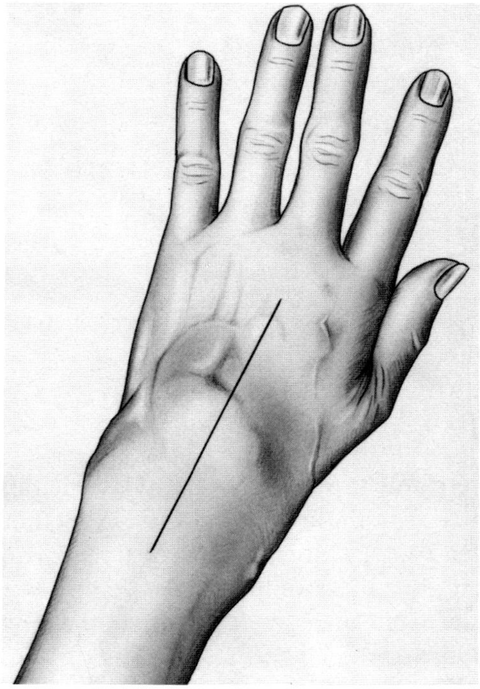

Fig. 1. Dorsal approach to the wrist by Mannerfelt [9].

At present, one can only speculate whether this might be a reason for the frequent radial deviation of the wrist. This deviation is certainly facilitated by the synovitis of the wrist itself which is, according to Pahle and Raunio [12], Mannerfelt [9] and Shapiro [17], one of the main causes for the ulnar deviation of the four long fingers.

Therefore we take the indication for a dorsal tenosynovectomy to be given whenever the conservative measures fail to achieve a restitution within a short period of time. This is particularly important since an operation gives relief of the pain and swelling, helps to avoid the rupture of the dorsal tendons along with all the complications of reconstruction, and decreases the subsequent impact on all the joints of the affected hand. From the technical point of view, we prefer the operative procedure that has been published by Gschwend [6] using the ap-

2 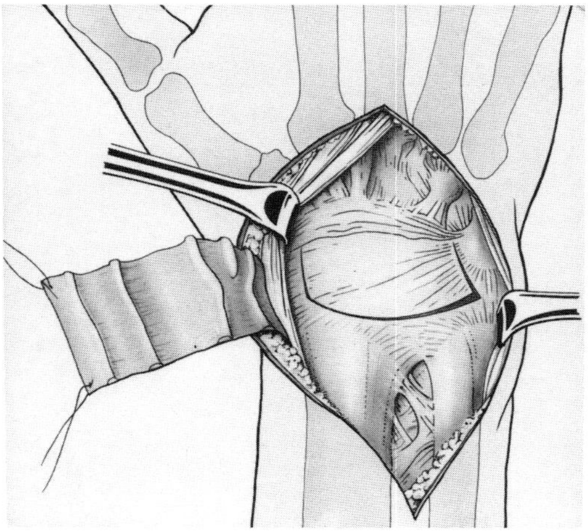 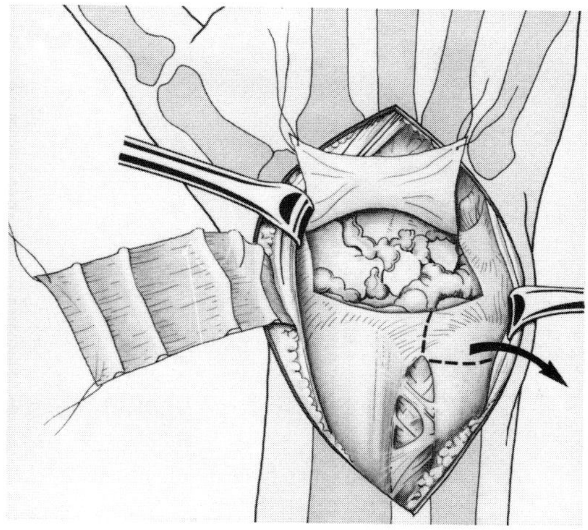 3

Fig. 2. Typical incision for synovectomy of the wrist.
Fig. 3. Synovitis of the wrist itself before synovectomy.

proach described by Mannerfelt [9] (fig. 1). When using this approach, a cautious resection of the head of the ulna including a synovectomy of the ulnar part of the wrist can be accomplished in the same session if a caput-ulna syndrome is present. Furthermore, this approach gives a good visual control even of the dorsal side of the wrist, thus allowing a full evaluation of it. If there is a slight suspicion of synovitis of the wrist itself, it will be incised in the typical way (fig. 2) and a synovectomy will be performed (fig. 3). We also would like to emphasize at this point the positive value of this procedure.

In the case of a luxation of the carpus to the volar side, a stabilization can be achieved together with the dorsal tenosynovectomy during the same session and using the same approach. As an alternative to the arthrodesis or alloarthroplasty we prefer the resection and interposition arthroplasty.

We should like to mention that in the cases of spontaneous ruptures of the dorsal tendons, the operative reconstruction is conducted during the same operation. In all these cases we use a coupling to the non-ruptured tendons if that is possible.

Table I. Dorsal tenosynovectomy of the wrist in rheumatoid arthritis (n = 69; both sides 10)

Patients:	59	Women:	40	Men:	19
Age:	21–78	Average:	51		

Table II. Dorsal tenosynovectomy of the wrist in rheumatoid arthritis (n = 69)

Combined surgical management	
Resection of the head of the ulna	65
Synovectomy of the wrist	18
Resection and interposition arthroplasty	9
Reconstruction of dorsal tendon ruptures	7

During the time from August 1980 to August 1984, a dorsal tenosynovectomy was performed in 69 hands. In 10 cases the operation was necessary on both sides. The 59 patients consisted of 40 women and 19 men. The age at the time of the operation varied from 21 to 78 years, the average was 51 years (table I).

In combination with a tenosynovectomy and during the same session we were able to perform 65 resections of the head of the ulna including a synovectomy of the ulnar part of the wrist, 18 synovectomies of the wrist itself, 7 reconstructions of the dorsal tendons and 9 resection and interposition arthroplasties (table II).

Complications consisted of 2 solitary spontaneous ruptures on the tenth postoperative day during the phase of mobilization, in 1 case of the dorsal tendon D IV and in the other case of D V. In both cases a successful reconstruction was accomplished in a second session. As a cause for this complication, we found an insufficient cover of the distal stump of the ulna after the resection. Therefore, we should like to emphasize at this point the importance of a sufficient cover (table III).

In 7 cases a skin necrosis developed with only a minor impact on the wound healing. In 1 case we saw a deep infection which led to a

Table III. Dorsal tenosynovectomy of the wrist in rheumatoid arthritis (n = 69)

Complications	
Infection combined with necrosis of dorsal tendons	1
Necrosis of the skin	7
Rupture of dorsal tendon D IV 10 days postop. and D V respectively (successful reconstruction at second operation)	2

Table IV. Dorsal tenosynovectomy of the wrist in rheumatoid arthritis (n = 42; follow-up: 1–4 years; average: 2 years)

	Preoperative pain	Postoperative pain
None	–	25
Light	–	11
Medium	9	6
Severe	33	–

Table V. Dorsal tenosynovectomy of the wrist in rheumatoid arthritis (n = 42; follow-up: 1–4 years; average: 2 years)

	Preoperative swelling	Postoperative swelling
None	–	38
Light	–	4
Medium	12	–
Severe	30	–

necrosis of all the dorsal tendons and which could be managed only by a resection of the tendons. Due to additional internal medical problems it was impossible to conduct an operative reconstruction in the meantime.

Since all of our patients are treated in our orthopedic outpatient department on a regular basis, we were able to evaluate these cases for

Table VI. Dorsal tenosynovectomy and synovectomy of the wrist in rheumatoid arthritis (n = 16; follow-up for an average time of 2.5 years)

	Preoperative pain	Postoperative pain
None	–	7
Light	–	9
Medium	4	–
Severe	12	–

Table VII. Dorsal tenosynovectomy and synovectomy of the wrist in rheumatoid arthritis (n = 16; follow-up for an average time of 2.5 years)

	Preoperative swelling	Postoperative swelling
None	–	15
Light	–	1
Medium	2	–
Severe	14	–

a period of 1–4 years after the operation with the average period being 2 years.

At this point we want to present 42 wrists on which only a dorsal tenosynovectomy had been conducted. In 38 of these cases a resection of the head of the ulna and in 7 cases a reconstruction of the dorsal tendons had been included. As can be seen in the tables IV and V, the improvement of both the pain and the swelling was remarkable. The function remained the same in most cases and there were no further spontaneous ruptures in the meantime. Our case material shows no relapse.

Furthermore, we were interested in the results of a simultaneous tenosynovectomy and synovectomy of the wrist. Here we were able to evaluate 16 wrists at an average of 2.5 years after the operation. In these cases the positive impact on both pain and swelling, as depicted in the tables VI and VII, was also present. Likewise the influence on the motion was not remarkable. It is of special interest, and in contradiction to the investigations of Vahvanen and Pätiäla [20], that the X-ray findings showed a non-progressive course in 12 cases. In 4 cases there was even a widening of the articular space of the wrist joint, a regression of the erosions and a sclerosing of the subchondral region (fig. 4).

a 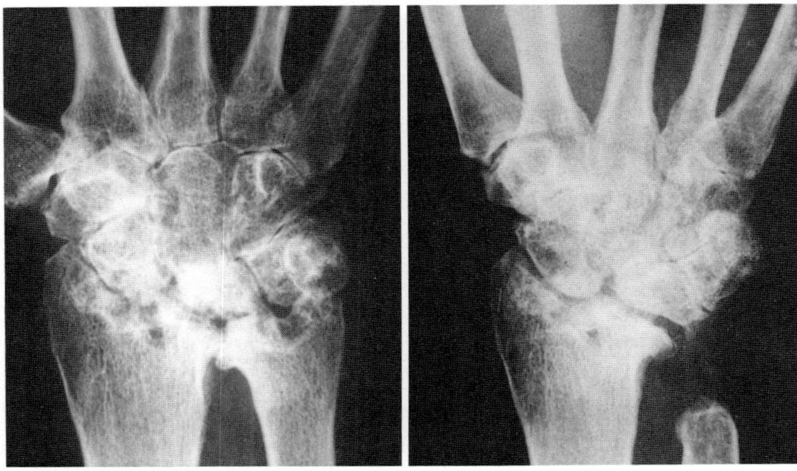 *b*

Fig. 4. H.E., female, 64 years. Rheumatoid arthritis. *a* Before and *b* 3 years after dorsal tenosynovectomy, resection of the ulna head and synovectomy of the wrist itself.

a 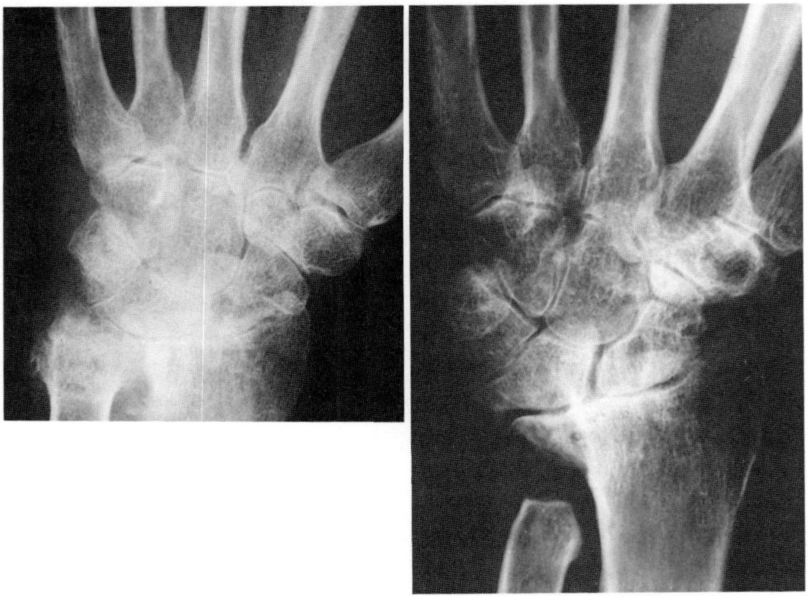 *b*

Fig. 5. H.G., male, 42 years. Rheumatoid arthritis. *a* Before and *b* 2.5 years after dorsal tenosynovectomy, resection of the ulna head and synovectomy of the wrist itself.

Table VIII. Dorsal tenosynovectomy and resection-interposition arthroplasty of the wrist in rheumatoid arthritis (n = 6; follow-up: 11–36 months)

Relief of pain with gain of power	5
Improving stability with better visual aspect	5
Average range of motion, degrees	30
Subjective results	
Good	5
Sufficient	1
Not sufficient	0

This was read as being a transition into a degenerative joint after rheumatoid arthritis. Subjectively the patients regarded themselves as being good in 9 cases and as being very good in 7 cases (fig. 5).

Finally, we should like to present the results of 6 hands in which a resection and interposition arthroplasty was conducted in the same session after a dorsal tenosynovectomy and a luxation of the carpus to the volar side. After a period of time of more than 30 months in 5 cases, and more than 11 months in 1 case, all cases showed complete pain relief and an increase of gross power.

The average range of motion was 30°. In 5 cases an improvement of the position and the shape of the wrist as well as a better stability was achieved. In 1 case the wrist shifted progressively to the ulnar side after the operation. In all cases the patients felt subjectively improved. Judged by the ability to handle the tasks of everyday life, the patients regarded the operative results as being good in 5 cases and as being sufficient in 1 case (table VIII).

Taking into account our results and emphasizing the importance of the preservation of the wrist motion for the whole hand, we can draw a similar conclusion as Howard [8] in 1955: Conducting an early dorsal tenosynovectomy and applying all the combination procedures necessary, there is little to lose, but much to be gained.

Summary

The results of our patients after dorsal tenosynovectomy in rheumatoid arthritis shows not only the positive influence of pain and swelling but also a prevention to spontaneous dorsal tendon ruptures.

By the same approach it is possible to combine other necessary surgical procedures, such as resection of the ulna head, reconstruction of dorsal tendons, synovectomy or resection-interposition arthroplasty of the wrist.

These patients with combined surgical management also show by 1–4 years after the operation a positive influence in pain and swelling. The range of motion of the wrist itself still remains the same.

References

1 Baeckdahl, M.: The caput ulnae syndrome in rheumatoid arthritis. Acta rheum. scand. suppl. 5 (1963).

2 Clayton, M.L.: Surgical treatment at the wrist in rheumatoid arthritis. J. Bone Jt Surg. *47:* 741 (1965).

3 Ehrlich, G.E.: The rheumatoid wrist. Am. Acad. gen. Practl. *35:* 78 (1967).

4 Fernandez-Pallazzi Vainio, K.: Synovectomy of the carpal joints in rheumatoid arthritis. A report of 47 cases. Archs interamer. Rheum. *8:* 249 (1965).

5a Flatt, A.E.: The care of the rheumatoid hand (Mosby, St. Louis 1963).

5b Flatt, A.E.: Care of the arthritic hand (Mosby, St. Louis 1983).

6 Gschwend, N.: Die operative Behandlung der chronischen Polyarthritis; 2. Aufl. (Thieme, Stuttgart 1977).

7 Hoos, R.; Refior, H.J.: Indikationskriterien zur Kombination von Tenosynovektomie und Synovektomie des Handgelenkes. Orth. Praxis *19:* 592 (1983).

8 Howard, L.D.: Surgical treatment of rheumatic tenosynovitis. J. Surg. A. *89:* 1163 (1955).

9a Mannerfelt, L.: Synovektomie der Strecksehnenfächer der Hand und des Handgelenkes Orthopädie *2:* 21 (1973).

9b Mannfelt, L.: Das unbehandelte rheumatische Handgelenk – natürliche Entwicklung und Verlauf. Akt. Rheumatol. *5:* 137 (1983).

10 Milford, L.: The hand; in Campbell, Operative orthopaedics. I, p. 264 (Mosby, St. Louis 1971).

11 Millander, L.H.; Nalebuff, N.: Preventive surgery – Tenosynovektomie and Synovektomie. Orthol. Clin. North Am. *6:* 765 (1975).

12 Pahle, J.A.; Raunio, P.: The influence of wrist position and finger deviation in the rheumatoid hand. J. Bone Jt Surg. *513:* 664 (1969).

13 Pulkki, T.: Rheumatoid deformities of the hand. Acta rheum. scand. *7:* 85 (1961).

14 Refior, H.J.; Baumann, D.: Ergebnisse der dorsalen Tenosynovektomie am Handgelenk. Akt. Rheumatol. *6:* 63 (1981).

15 Refior, H.J.: Synovektomie des Handgelenkes. Akt. Rheumatol. *8:* 157 (1983).

16 Refior, H.J.; et al.: Langzeitergebnisse nach Kniegelenkssynovektomie bei chronischer Polyarthritis. Z. Orthop. *417:* 13–20 (1979).

17 Shapiro, J.S.: The etiology of ulnar drift: a new factor. J. Bone Hand Surg. *50A:* 634 (1968).

18 Stellbrink, G.: Arthroplastik des Handgelenkes. Orthopädie *2:* 48 (1973).

19 Straub, L.R.; Ranawat, G.S.: The wrist in rheumatoid arthritis. J. Bone Hand Surg. *51H:* 1 (1969).

20 Yahvanen, V.; Pätiäla, H.: Synovektomy of the wrist in rheumatoid arthritis and related diseases. Archs Orthop. Trauma Surg. *102:* 230 (1984).

21 Wessinghage, D.; Miehlke, H.: Die Kniegelenkssynovektomie bei rheumatischen Erkrankungen und ihre Ergebnisse. Dt. med. Wschr. *15:* 685 (1970).

Prof. Dr. H.J. Refior, MD, Orthopädische Klinik
der Medizinischen Hochschule Hannover,
Postfach 61072, D-3000 Hannover 61 (FRG)

Rheumatology, vol. 11, pp. 49–55 (Karger, Basel 1987)

The Use of Power Staple Fixation in the Surgical Management of the Rheumatoid Hand and Wrist

Jules S. Shapiro

Rush Presbyterian-St. Luke's Medical Center, Chicago, Ill., USA

Introduction

Over the years, arthrodesis, arthroplasty, tendon repairs and transfers and synovectomy have all contributed to gains in functional capacity for the rheumatoid patient.

Today, demands for maximal return on monies spent on health care have placed even greater emphasis upon which combinations of surgical procedures can be performed safely and effectively to restore such function.

Hastings [1], reporting to the American Society for Surgery of the Hand in 1984, noted that multiple simultaneous procedures were well tolerated in the reconstruction of the rheumatoid hand and wrist without causing significant alterations in complication rate, postoperative course, and final results from that expected from multiple staged reconstructive procedures. This differs from the way most rheuma surgeons have learned and practice reconstructive surgery; namely, procedures to be performed at any one sitting should be limited and staged.

In attempting to reconcile maximal procedures with achieving optimal functional return, a new (and yet very old) type of fixation has been used for the past 1.5 years.

Staples have been and are presently used in many orthopedic applications. The literature lists several references yearly [2–5] to their use for bone fixation. However, their use has been limited primarily because of difficulty in insertion and because of a reputation for poor holding power.

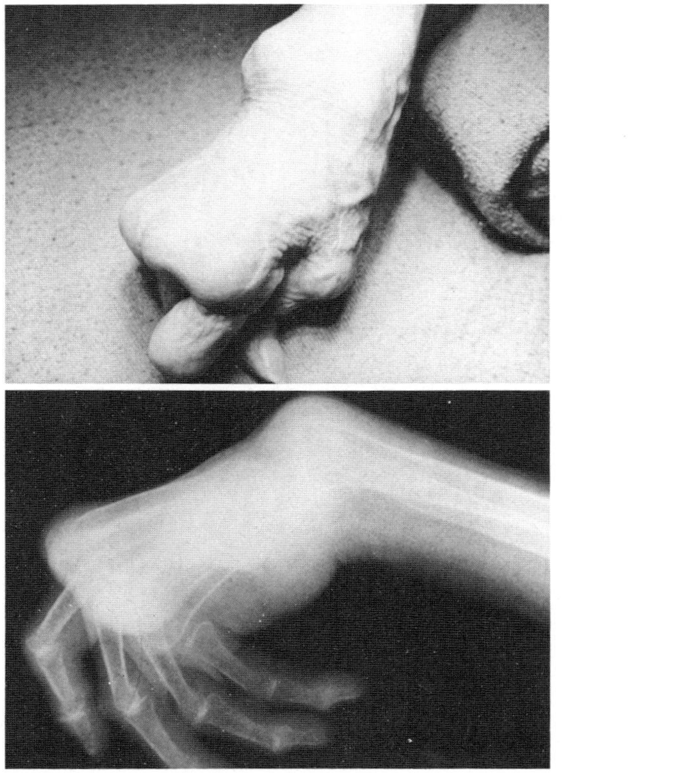

a

b

c

d

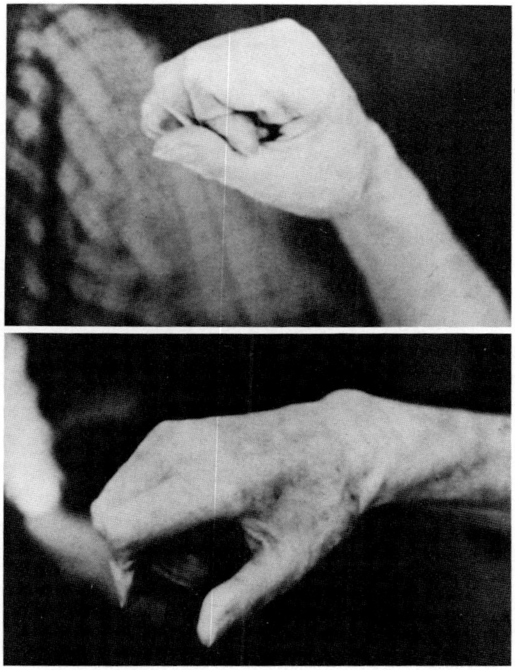

e

Fig. 1. M.B., 69-year-old female with severe involvement hand and wrist. *a* Preoperative photograph. *b* Preoperative X-ray. *c* X-Ray of thumb interphalangeal arthrodesis, 17 months postoperatively. *d* X-Ray of wrist 17 months postoperatively. *e* Photographs of hand 17 months after surgery.

By converting them from a poor holding device to an efficient fixator, we have been able to use staples in new areas never before thought as being amenable for their usage.

The conversion has been achieved by the addition of a guided, reproducible power source for driving the staple, a 'staple-gun'. This has resulted in easier technique with savings of operative time, and therefore has allowed more procedures to be performed safely at one time, but more importantly, has resulted in the ability to start rehabilitative activity earlier than previously thought possible for certain procedures.

Materials and Methods

From December 1983, through May 1985, this type of fixation was used over 50 times for a variety of orthopedic indications. In 26 hands and wrists in 20 rheumatoid arthritic patients, it has been used as follows:

Six times as fixation for fusion of the interphalangeal (IP) joint of the thumb, once for supplemental fixation for arthrodesis of the metacarpophalangeal (MCP) joint of the thumb, once for fixation after osteotomy at the wrist, 8 times for supplemental fixation of total wrist arthrodesis, and 10 times for limited wrist arthrodesis.

Usage was divided into two basic groups: (1) the severely handicapped, where multiple procedures are of profound benefit, and (2) in the moderately involved rheumatoid wrist, where a new set of procedures appears most promising.

An example of the former was M.B., a 69-year-old female with a 20-year history of rheumatoid arthritis (fig. 1). At the time of surgery in December 1983, her hand function had deteriorated significantly. Her general medical condition dictated that as many procedures as would be benificial be done at one sitting. Consequently, the following was performed: wrist arthrodesis, Darrach resection, dorsal tenosynovectomy; arthroplasty of MCP 1–5 with transfer of EPL to base of proximal phalanx, and arthrodesis of the IP joint of the thumb (all performed within a single tourniquet time of approximately 2 h and 15 min).

Power staples were used as solitary fixation for the IP joint and for supplemental fixation at the wrist. Rehabilitation was started as usual, but thumb function begun after 2 weeks of immobilization for the tendon transfer. No attempt was made to restrict pinch or grasp. At 2 years after surgery, the patient was functioning well with all operative sites functioning as expected. In other thumb arthrodeses, without tendon transfers, no immobilization is used and activity is started at day three after surgery.

Having now performed this combination of procedures many times, we feel confidence that it works well and does not compromise the patient's extremity.

We have also used staple fixation for thumb MCP arthrodeses, and now perform the operation either together with multiple procedures or as a solitary outpatient procedure. The most exciting application of this fixation has been in limited wrist arthrodesis. Building on the works of Crosby et al. [6] and Watson et al. [7] in the degenerative wrist, and Nalebuff and Garrod [8] and particularly Chamay et al. [9] in the rheumatoid, limited arthrodesis has opened new therapeutic ground in the vast area which always lay between carpal synovectomy and more radical procedures.

Rationale behind limited arthrodesis is simple. Patients who spontaneously ankylose at the radiolunate joint usually retain some satisfactory wrist motion, but no longer risk transmigration of the carpus ulnarward. Their finger deformities also do not appear to have the zigzag collapse associated with either radial wrist rotation or ulnar wrist transmigration. The question arose as to whether surgically creating this condition could result in maintaining motion at the other intercarpal joints as well?

Authors performing limited wrist arthrodesis, using either k-wires, screws, etc., have advocated a minimum of 6 weeks immobilization. This results in limited motion and necessity for removal of the k-wires at a later date. While still using at least 6 weeks immobilization in degenerative joint disease, we have reduced immobilization to only 3 weeks after such procedures in the rheumatoid.

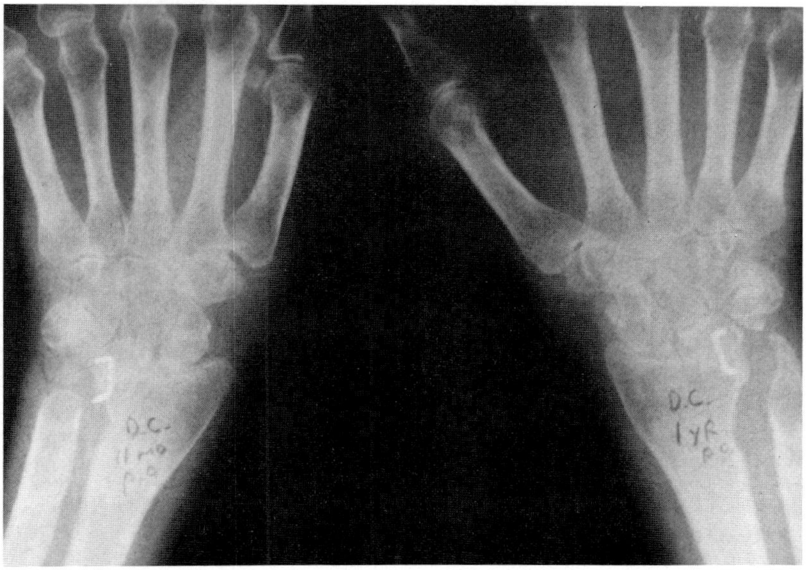

a

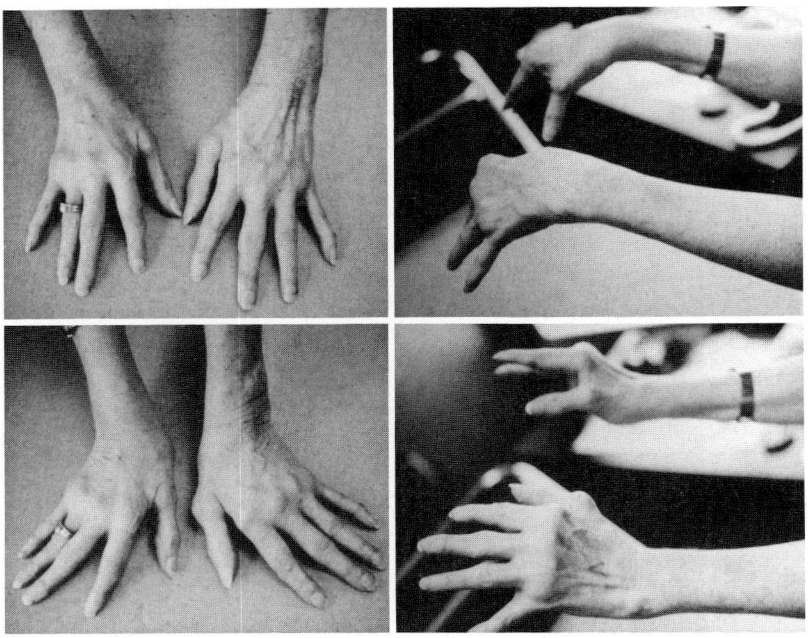

b

Fig. 2. D.C., 43-year-old female. *a* X-Ray of both wrists 11 and 12 months after bilateral radio/lunate arthrodesis. *b* Range of motion of wrists at 1 year after surgery.

Rheumatoid limited wrist arthrodesis using power staple fixation was performed 12 times over the same time period; 5 radio/lunate, 3 radio/scapho/lunate, and one each scapho/lunate and scapho/luno/capitate.

An example is D.C., a 43-year-old female with a history of rheumatoid arthritis of 5 years duration (fig. 2). She underwent radio/lunate arthrodesis of her right wrist in June 1984 and of her left wrist in July 1984. Her X-rays at 11 and 12 months postoperatively show excellent evidence that surgical intervention has indeed created such a radio-lunate fusion, while still retaining good wrist motion.

Limited wrist arthrodesis using this fixation has many advantages. First, it provides the opportunity to correct the tendency for ulnar/volar transmigration of the carpus. Second, it mimics a course found naturally in some patients who maintain considerable wrist function. Third, it fills the therapeutic void between the procedure recommended for the patient considered beyond synovectomy and too good for total arthrodesis or arthroplasty. And lastly, it is what Soutter [10] described as 'a winner'; namely an operation which is likely to tax the patient only minimally and at the same time virtually guarantee, from the symptomatic or functional point of view, to be a winner. The power staple has proven to be very valuable in obtaining these ends.

Conclusion

It is believed that power stable fixation is likely to play an ever-increasing role in the reconstruction of the rheumatoid hand and wrist.

Summary

Application of a power source for insertion of staples greatly expands their applicability. Their usefulness in the surgery of the rheumatoid hand is described as used by the author over a 1.5-year period. Its applications have included multiple procedures for the severely handicapped and limited wrist arthrodesis in the earlier stages of the disease. Its advantages over more conventional types of fixation are delineated.

References

1 Hasting, H.: Evaluation of the efficacy of single-stage reconstruction for multiple joint level rheumatoid deformity. 39th Annu. Meet. Am. Soc. Surg. Hand, Atlanta 1984.

2 Benneddache, Y.; Gottesman, H.; Fourrier, P.: Multiple stapling for wrist arthrodesis in the nonrheumatoid patient. J. Hand Surg. *9A:* 256–261 (1984).

3 Burkus, J.K.; Moore, D.W.; Raykroft, J.F.: Valgus deformity of the ankle in myelodysplastic patients. Correction by stapling of the medial part of the distal tibial physis. J. Bone Jt Surg. *65A:* 1157–1162 (1983).

4 Yde, J.; Kristensen, K.D.: Inferior tibio-fibular diastasis treated by staple fixation. J. Trauma *21:* 483–485 (1981).
5 Sailer, H.F.: Osteosynthesis of orbital margin fractures via the transconjuctival approach using staples. J. Maxillofac. Surg. *5:* 184–186 (1977).
6 Crosby, E.B.; Linscheid, R.; Dobyns, J.: Scaphotrapezial trapezoidal arthrosis. J. Hand Surg. *3:* 223–234 (1978).
7 Watson, H.K.; Goodman, M.L.; Johnson, T.R.: Limited wrist arthrodesis. II. Intercarpal and radiocarpal combinations. J. Hand Surg. *6:* 223–233 (1981).
8 Nalebuff, E.A.; Garrod, K.J.: Present approach to the severely involved rheumatoid wrist. Orthop. Clin. North Am. *15:* 369–380 (1984).
9 Chamay, A.; Della Santa, D.; Vilaseca, A.: Radiolunate arthrodesis, factor of stability for the rheumatoid wrist. Ann. Chir. Main *2:* 5–17 (1983).
10 Souter, W.A.: Planning treatment of the rheumatoid hand. Hand *11:* 3–11 (1979).

Jules S. Shapiro, MD, 1725 W. Harrison Street, Suite 492, Chicago, IL 60612 (USA)

Rheumatology, vol. 11, pp. 56–58 (Karger, Basel 1987)

The Function of the Hand after Surgical Treatment of the MP Joints in Rheumatoid Arthritis – A Comparative Study

R. Siorpaes, F. Kerschbaumer

Department of Orthopaedic Surgery, University of Innsbruck
(Head: Prof. R. Bauer), Innsbruck, Austria

Introduction

The purpose of the follow-up examination at issue was the assessment of the influence of both the synovectomy and the metacarpophalangeal (MP) arthroplasty onto the function of the hand after a medium-term observation period. We were looking for limiting factors for one of the said operations.

Method of Examination

After an average observation period of 5 years 59 patients were examined again. Of a total of 186 operated MP joints there were 95 synovectomies and 91 arthroplasties, 81 of them Swanson spacer. The average age of the patients at the time of operation was 52.3 years. With the exception of eight of them, all patients were suffering from seropositive arthritis and, on an average, had been showing the symptoms of that disorder for 12.5 years. The following parameters of examination were employed: the preoperative flexibility was compared with the flexibility at the time of the follow-up examination. Investigations regarding dexterity were made by questionnaires including inquiries about daily activities.

In our opinion, indications for an MP synovectomy are therapy-resistant swelling and pain for a period of more than one half year, and Larsen stages 0, 1 and 2, in some cases even 3. In the event of higher Larsen stages or severe deformities MP arthroplasties were made. Patients with additional operations were excluded from the examination.

Results

MP Synovectomies. Of 37 synovectomized patients only one reported an equal amount of pain as during the preoperative state. All other patients showed a considerable improvement of their symptoms of pain. The examination of the strength of the various fingers with the intrinsicmeter showed that as opposed to the preoperative state the strength had almost doubled. On an average, the preoperative range of movement was 81°. The postoperative range of movement had decreased by an average of 20°.

19 joints showed an increase in their range of movement. These joints were exclusively in the Larsen stages 1 and 2. Loss of range of movement: the fourth and fifth fingers were affected more severely, while the second finger showed even an improvement in its range of movement in all cases. The subjective assessment of the dexterity based on the questionnaire ranged at an almost unchanged preoperative 76% and postoperative 70%.

MP Arthroplasties. With these operations, too, a distinct alleviation of pain was achieved, i.e. by an average of one point on the four-part pain scale. There was no marked increase in the strength of the various fingers after the MP arthroplasties (preoperative 1.8, postoperative 2.1).

As opposed to the preoperative state the range of movement showed a definite decrease. Average values range at 15°; the fourth and fifth finger again showed even poorer movement. After the MP arthroplasties the dexterity of the patients was pronouncedly improved, namely by 23% or almost one quarter.

Discussion

MP synovectomy resulted in a reduction of pain in virtually all cases. The fact that the strength had almost doubled, most likely is a result of this decrease of pain. Even though the range of movement had decreased and the disorder progressed, dexterity had remained unchanged on the whole. This fact, as well as the circumstance that with none of the synovectomized fingers a severe deformity had occurred within the 5 years under review, strongly stresses the prophylactic character of this operation.

Despite of a reduced range of movement and a merely slight increase of strength the joints treated with Swanson spacer showed a better function, i.e. by one quarter. This may be deduced from the fact that the fingers were in a more functional range afterwards.

In the course of analyzing the unsatisfactory results we noted that the patients complaining about restricted function, i.e. patients with synovectomized as well as arthroplastized joints, usually showed a restricted range of movement of the proximal interphalangeal (PIP) joint, as well. The joints treated with arthroplasty, in particular, were adversely influenced by that circumstance and showed worse results. For us this is reason enough to pay closer attention to the PIP joint in future surgical treatment on the one hand, and - on the other hand - not to place too high hopes in the functional result if the PIP joints are in bad shape.

Summary

After an average observation period of 5 years 186 metacarpophalangeal (MP) joints with synovectomies or arthroplasties were subjected to a follow-up examination. Regarding MP synovectomies nearly all patients showed a considerable improvement of their symptoms of pain. The postoperative state of strength had almost doubled, while a loss of movement of an average of 20° was observed. The fourth and fifth finger were affected more severely. The subjective assessment of the dexterity remained unchanged from the preoperative to the postoperative stage. MP arthroplasties led to a decrease of pain, an increase of strength, and a loss of the range of movement, but also to an increase of the dexterity of almost one quarter. One reason for bad results were proximal interphalangeal joints in poor shape.

Dr. Robert Siorpaes, Department of Orthopaedic Surgery,
University of Innsbruck, Anichstrasse 35, A-6020 Innsbruck (Austria)

Rheumatology, vol. 11, pp. 59–63 (Karger, Basel 1987)

Vainio's Metacarpophalangeal Arthroplasty

A Material of 42 Rheumatoid Hands

Vappu Uuspää

Rheumatism Foundation Hospital, Hamina, Finland

Introduction

Painful, destructed metacarpophalangeal joints are an everyday problem in rheumatoid surgery. Several methods of reconstruction have been presented. Vainio's metacarpophalangeal arthroplasty has been used for more than 20 years. In Vainio's arthroplasty the metacarpal heads is resected and the extensor tendon is used as interposition material. Thus, the extensor tendon is shortened, flexors are not. Large resection and thorough intrinsic release may result in the metacarpophalangeal hyperextension position that interferes with the hand's function.

Patients and Methods

38 patients: 30 F, age 24–71, mean 51, and 8 M, age 33–63, mean 51. 26 unemployable, 9 light manual/sedentary work, 1 heavy manual work, 2 housewives.

Rheumatoid disease: 33 rheumatoid arthritis, 4 JCA, 1 LED, all polyarthritic, had continued 5–46 years, mean 18 years. ESR ranged from 5 to 125, mean 43. CRP was positive in 21. 42 hands, 25 R, 17 L, had been involved 4–46 years, mean 17 years.

Previous operations of the hand-wrist area: 9 metacarpophalangeal (MCP) synovectomy; 4 Straub transposition; 3 abductor digiti minimi tenotomy; 2 Vainio arthroplasty, 2nd to 3rd and 2nd MCP joint; 1 3rd and 5th extensor tendon reconstruction; 1 EIP transposition; 3 proximal interphalangeal (PIP) synovectomy; 3 PIP arthrodesis; 6 digital flexor tenosynovectomy; 5 volar carpal tenosynovectomy; 4 dorsal carpal tenosynovectomy/carpal synovectomy; 24 carpal arthrodesis; 5 thumb MCP arthrodesis; 2 interphalangeal (IP) pollicis arthrodesis; 2 EPL reconstruction; 1 MCP pollicis synovectomy; 1 IP pollicis synovectomy; 1 CMC pollicis synovectomy; 1 traumatic amputation of the ring and little fingers; 4 hands had not been operated on before arthroplasty.

Medical treatment at the time of the arthroplasty: 15 gold; 10 penicillamine; 4 antimalarial; 19 glucocorticoids; 16 salicylates; 17 indomethacin; 22 other 'rheuma' medicines.

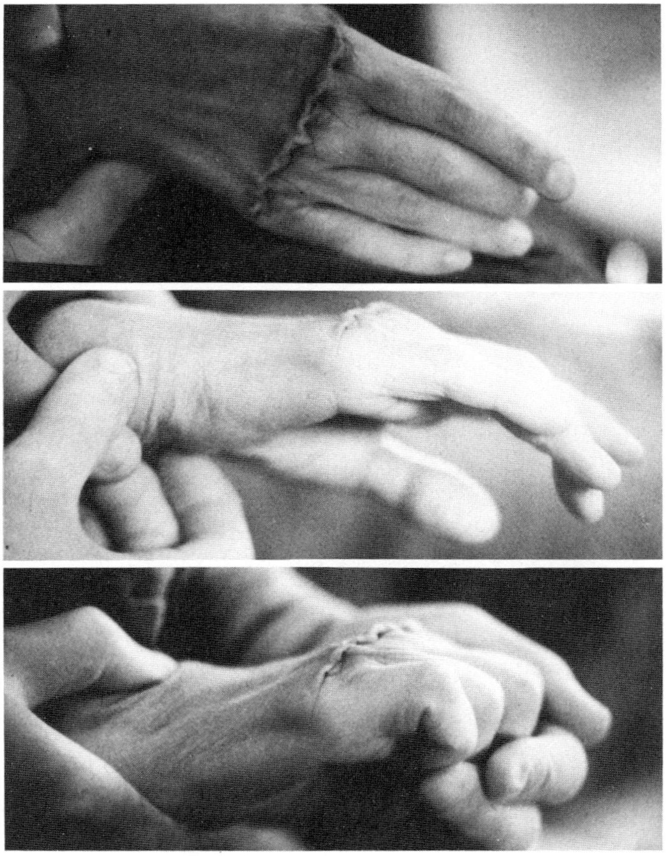

Fig. 1. See text.

Arthroplasties were performed by one surgeon during the years 1978–84. In 37 hands all four MCP joints were operated on. In 2 hands 2nd to 4th MCP joints, in one hand 3rd to 5th, in 1 hand 2nd to 3rd, and in one hand the 4th MCP joint was operated on.

A transverse dorsal incision was used. At first abductor digiti minimi was released, and synovectomy of the MCP joints was done.

To prevent MCP hyperextension position and ulnar deviation the metacarpal head were only partially resected, the osteotomies sloping radially and volarly leaving the ulnar collateral intact. The radial collateral was reattached somewhat more proximally and dorsally with slight radial overcorrection. From the 27th hand on, at first only at the 2nd and 3rd MCP joints the extensor tendon was fixed with an extra suture to the radial remnants of the extensor hood and capsula on the metacarpal head leaving the MCP joints in slight flexion allowing PIP flexion to about 90° peroperatively (fig. 1).

If extensor tendons were fixed in previous dorsal carpal scar tissue, the extensor tendons were left slacker to allow proper MCP flexion. In four hands Straub transposition was done. Postoperative compression bandage was removed on the 5th to 7th postoperative days. Active training in a dynamic splint was started, and a night splint to prevent ulnar drift was worn until at 6 weeks normal use of the hand was encouraged.

In 19 hands other operations were performed during the same session: 10 MCP pollicis arthrodesis; 4 MCP pollicis synovectomy; 3 IP pollicis arthrodesis; 1 IP pollicis synovectomy; 2 CMC pollicis arthroplasty with ECRL interposition; 1 adductor release; 2 5th MCP synovectomy; 1 3rd PIP synovectomy; 1 VY extensor tenoplasty of the 4th PIP joint; 3 excisions of subcutaneous nodes.

Results

34 hands with 131 operated MCP joints were re-examined 6 months to 6 years 10 months after arthroplasty. Average follow-up was 2 years 5 months. There was tendency to palmar subluxation with flexion contracture up to 60° (one finger), average 10°. 15% of the fingers were in the hyperextended position, up to 55°, most commonly the little finger, 10 cases, and the ring finger, 7 cases. Range of flexion was 40° on average, range 0–90°. Peroperative radial overcorrection tended to disappear (fig. 2, 3). 11% of the fingers deviated radially 5–15° (one case with previous EIP transposition).

On maximal active extension 30% of the fingers deviated ulnarly 5–35°, average 15°. In one hand with Straub transposition the fingers deviated radially 5° each, in other hands there was no MCP deviation. Neither earlier MCP synovectomy (8 hands) nor carpal arthrodesis (9 hands without other previous operations) worsened the average result, as to flexion contracture, range of flexion, or MCP deviation. 75% of these wrist fusion cases had the fingers in 0-position, 22% deviated ulnarly, 14% radially.

Other operations of the same hand in the same session did not worsen the result (16 hands). In 8 hands there was some irritation of the operative wound or around the sutures: in 2 hands of one patient *Staphylococcus epidermidis* was cultured. In others the cultures were negative. 6 of these hands were re-examined: the average range of flexion was 50° and only one finger deviated ulnarly, and 4 fingers hyperextended 10–35°. In 2 hands the volar subluxation caused inconvenience in heavy manual work: in 1 hand the proximal phalanx of the index finger, in the other that of the middle finger, was bulging palmarly.

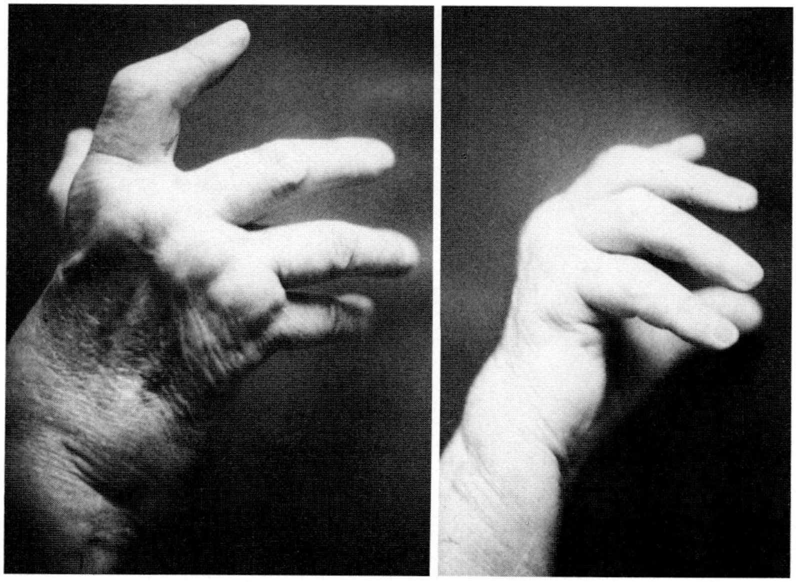

Fig. 2. A female patient, age 57, former hospital aid. LED 15 years. Hand involved 15 years. Carpal arthrodesis 1 year previously. Preoperative flexion contracture.

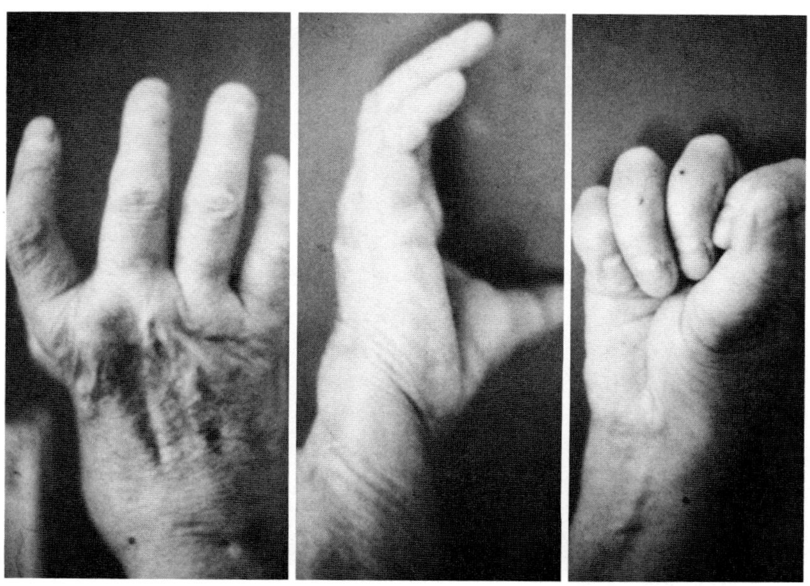

Fig. 3. Same patient. Postoperative result.

Discussion

Vainio's MCP arthroplasty is a sound method that uses extensor tendon as interposition material. Nevertheless, extensor tendon shortening interferes with extensor flexor balance and carries the risk of the MCP hyperextension position.

In the present material a trial to counteract the hyperextension tendency was done at first by limited resection, volarly sloping osteotomy planes, which was not enough to prevent the deformity. Radial fixation of the extensor tendon was added. The resulting tendency to palmar subluxation usually did not disturb function nor cosmetic appearance. The average range of flexion was the same as with the original method. Severe PIP joint flexion contracture seems to contribute in inducing the hyperextension deformity.

Summary

Vainio's metacarpophalangeal arthroplasty was performed on 42 rheumatoid hands, 25 R, 17 L, of 38 patients: 8 male, age 33–63, mean 51, and 30 female, age 24–71, mean 51, by one surgeon during the years 1978–84.

In order to prevent the metacarpophalangeal hyperextension position, the most common complication of Vainio arthroplasty, and ulnar deviation: (1) Metacarpal heads were only partially resected, the osteotomies sloping radially and volarwards, leaving the ulnar collaterals intact, and reattaching the radial collateral with slight radial overcorrection. (2) The extensor tendon was fixed to the radial remnants of the capsula and the extensor hood leaving the metacarpophalangeal joints in slight flexion.

The result was tendency to palmar subluxation and flexion contracture of the metacarpophalangeal joints, 10° on average, and range of flexion 40° on average, from 0 to 90°. 15% of the fingers were in the hyperextended position, up to 55°. On maximal active extension 30% of the fingers deviated ulnarly 5–35°, average 15°; 11% deviated radially 5–15°.

References

Raunio, P.: Die Arthroplastik der MCP-Gelenke in der rheumatoiden Arthritis. Orthopädie *2:* 42–43 (1973).

Vainio, K.; Reiman, J.; Pulkki, T.: Results of arthroplasty of the MCP joints in RA. WiederherstChir. Traumat. *9:* 1–7 (1967).

Vappu Uuspää, MD, Rheumatism Foundation Hospital, Murtalhontie 279,
SF-49420 Hamina 2 (Finland)

Rheumatology, vol. 11, pp. 64–70 (Karger, Basel 1987)

MCP Arthroplasty in RA

Comparison of Vainio and Swanson Techniques

M. Hämäläinen, H. Raemy

Rheumatism Foundation Hospital, Heinola, Finland

Several allo- and autoarthroplasty techniques have been introduced for the treatment of rheumatic destruction and deformities at the metacarpophalangeal (MCP) joint level. Very naturally, Vainio's excision tendon interposition arthroplasty has been extensively used in Heinola, in the hospital where the technique was designed. Since 1976, silastic excision implant technique by Swanson has been in concomitant use.

No definite indications have been specified for the use of one or the other of these arthroplasties, but choice of technique has been more or less random. Therefore, it seemed reasonable to compare the results of these two arthroplasties in rather identical materials operated upon in the same hospital by the same surgeons. Very unfortunately, no prospective follow-up regimens were in use, but the study was retrospective.

Material (table I)

The matching criteria were as follows: same sex; same age; same hand and, if possible, same joint; same date of operation ± 6 months.

From the time period 1976–78 we were able to collect 32 matched pairs of patients, one series with Vainio's arthroplasty, the other series with Swanson, altogether 80 operated joints in each. The series were statistically similar, except for sex and age, as well concerning diagnosis, duration of general disease and local symptoms. A rather wide variation was revealed between patients regarding preoperative grip power, but still the series were similar (table II). At the time of surgery, only minor differences were found in medication. On standard radiographs, ap- and side views, the destruction grade from 0

Table I. MCP arthroplasty: Vainio vs Swanson. 32 patients in each series (28 females; 4 males)

	Vainio	Swanson
Age: mean, years	44.3	44.2
range, years	18–66	20–66
Diagnosis sero positive RA	20	18
sero negative RA	6	9
JCP	6	5
Duration of:		
Systemic disease, years	6–45	4–38
Local symptoms, years	2–43	2–38

Table II. MCP arthroplasties: Vainio vs Swanson. Grip power ($kp/cm^2 \times 10$) preoperative

	Vainio patients	Swanson patient
0	1	8
0–10	9	6
11–20	13	10
21–30	7	6
31–	2	2

χ^2: $p < 0.02$.

to 5 according to Larsen was assessed, and mutual congruence of metacarpal bone and basic phalanx was measured. The series were statistically similar in this concern (table III). Very unfortunately, accurate and reliable preoperative measurements of mobility as well as lateral deviations were missing. Follow-up averaged 3.2 years (range 2.0–5.5 years).

Results

Early Complications. Only in two Swanson hands were wound-healing problems met, with no long-term effect, however. Bone and prosthetic changes do not belong to the scope of this study, because the

Table III. MCP arthroplasties: Vainio vs Swanson. Preoperative radiological grading

Grade (0–5)	Vainio	Swanson
0	–	–
1	–	–
2	–	–
3	10	6
4	7	14
5	63	60

χ^2: $p < 0.1$.

Table IV. MCP arthroplasties: Vainio vs Swanson. Postoperative pain

	Vainio	Swanson
1 nil	56	64
2 slight	20	8
3 pronounced	4	8
4 severe	–	–

χ^2: $p < 0.01$.

principles of procedures are so different that their comparison here is not relevant.

Pain (table IV). Pain evaluation joint by joint does not give much evidence about one or the other technique's superiority. There were more totally painfree joints in the Swanson series, not statistically significant, however.

Range of Movement (table V). Active total range of movement (ROM) averaged nearly equally: 43.7° in the Swanson series and 45.3° in the Vainio series. After Vainio arthroplasty, however, there was a

Table V. MCP arthroplasties: Vainio (V) vs Swanson (S). ROM at FU; degree, mean

		Active	Passive
MCP II	S	16.1 – 52.3	-5.0 – 62.0
	V	-0.7 – 48.3	-30.7 – 62.9
MCP II	S	12.5 – 58.8	-7.9 – 67.5
	V	0.5 – 44.1	-27.5 – 57.2
MCP III	S	7.9 – 52.9	-14.7 – 61.5
	V	-5.0 – 37.7	-36.1 – 55.0
MCP IV	S	6.5 – 54.7	-16.9 – 61.6
	V	-17.5 – 28.9	-46.0 – 39.6
MCP V	S	10.8 – 54.5	-11.1 – 63.2
	V	-0.6 – 39.7	-35.0 – 53.6
Total	S	10.8 – 54.5	-11.1 – 63.2
	V	-5.6 – 39.7	-35.0 – 53.6

Minus figures of extension indicate hyperextension.

Table VI. MCP arthroplasties: Vainio vs Swanson. Postoperative grip power

	Vainio	Swanson
Less than preop.	15	12
Same as preop.	5	4
Better than preop.	12	16

χ^2: n.s.

tendency to hyperextension, and correspondingly flexion limited to about 40°. Passively, Vainio joints presented even more instability as hyperextension reached a value of 35.0° compared with 11.1° in the Swanson series. The mobility of separate joints varied slightly, but in the same proportion in both series.

Table VII. MCP arthroplasties: Vainio vs Swanson. Postoperative swelling and deformities

		Vainio	Swanson	Statistics χ^2
Swelling	1 nil	64	64	
	2 slight	16	12	$p < 0.05$
	3 pronounced	–	4	
Ulnar subluxation	1	40	48	
	2	16	24	$p < 0.01$
	3	24	8	
Volar subluxation	1	36	72	
	2	24	4	$p < 0.001$
	3	20	4	
Ulnar deviation	0–10°	24	36	
	11–20°	16	16	$p < 0.02$
	21–30°	12	16	
	>31°	12	4	
Radial deviation	0–10°	8	4	n.t.
	11–20°	8	4	

Grip Power (table VI). Fifteen patients out of 32 lost in grip power in the Vainio series, but for twelve patients the procedure improved the above. In the Swanson series, assessment gave a slightly better figure, not statistically significant, however.

Swelling (table VII). Both techniques were equally good in decreasing swelling.

Congruence and Correction of Deformities. Silastic implant, although soft and flexible, seems to give better stability and mutual congruence, while expressed as ulnar or volar subluxation of basic phalanx. When assessing ulnar deviation, which is the most frequent in rheumatoid arthritis (RA), the difference between series is not that obvious any more.

Table VIII. MCP arthroplasties: Vainio (V) vs Swanson (S). Functional state at FU

Grade	Right (n = 43/45)				Left (n = 37/35)			
	1	2	3	4	1	2	3	4
	V S	V S	V S	V S	V S	V S	V S	V S
MCP II	3 / 6	4 / 4	2 / 3	3 / 0	5 / 3	5 / 4	0 / 0	2 / 3
III	4 / 7	2 / 4	2 / 3	3 / 0	6 / 3	3 / 4	0 / 1	2 / 1
IV	3 / 3	2 / 3	2 / 3	2 / 0	3 / 5	2 / 3	0 / 0	2 / 1
V	2 / 3	3 / 4	3 / 2	3 / 0	3 / 3	2 / 2	0 / 0	2 / 1
Percent	28 / 42 n.s.	25 / 33 n.s.	22 / 25 n.s.	25 / 0 $p < 0.001$	46 / 40 n.s.	33 / 40 n.s.	0 / 3 n.s.	21 / 17 n.s.

1 = Marked improvement; 2 = slight improvement; 3 = same as preoperative; 4 = worse.

Function at Follow-Up (table VIII). Despite some differences that were seen in separate analyses, patients' subjective assessment of the functional ability was similar in both series.

Satisfaction. The same thing as above can be shown by the figures about patients' compliance to the operation. 84% in both series would like to have the operation again.

Discussion

Vainio's arthroplasty is certainly more complicated and technically challenging than Swanson's technique. Possibly the surgeons in Heinola are more familiar with the technical details of the resection tendon interposition technique than the people on average. Further, the important finesses in the Swanson technique have not been accomplished in a proper way. Results have to be evaluated against this background. We did not evaluate the amount and significance of shortening of fingers which is a result after Vainio's arthroplasty. Possibly the matter has more or less cosmetic meaning only.

Conclusions

Although some differences were found between the series regarding pain relief, ROM, stability and deformity correction, both arthroplasties gave similar results regarding patients' satisfaction. In the light of the present series, Vainio's excision tendon interposition technique still seems to have place in some selected cases. In the case of severe bone destruction autoarthroplasty has to be considered instead of the implant technique.

References

Hellum, C.; Vainio, K.: Arthroplasty of the metacarpophalangeal joints in rheumatoid arthritis with transposition of the interosseous muscles. Scand. J. plast. reconstr. Surg. *2:* 139–142 (1968).

Raunio, P.: Arthroplastik der MCP-Gelenke in der rheumatoiden Arthritis. Orthopäde *2:* 42–43 (1973).

Swanson, A.B.: Surgery of established rheumatoid deformities in hand; in Cruess, Mitchell, Surgery of rheumatoid arthritis, pp. 177–198 (Lippincott, Philadelphia 1971).

Vainio, K.: Surgery of rheumatoid arthritis; in Cooper, The craft of surgery, pp. 1809–1830 (Little, Brown, Boston 1964).

M. Hämäläinen, MD, Rheumatism Foundation Hospital, Rautsalo C 9,
SF–18100 Heinola 10 (Finland)

Rheumatology, vol. 11, pp. 71–79 (Karger, Basel 1987)

Implant Arthroplasty of the Metacarpophalangeal Joints in Rheumatoid Arthritis

Veijo Vahvanen, Timo Viljakka

The Orthopaedic Hospital of the Invalid Foundation, Helsinki, Finland

In rheumatoid arthritis (RA) the metacarpophalangeal joints (MP) are frequently destroyed. Resection arthroplasties [1–3] or replacement arthroplasties [4–7] are the main methods used to correct severe deformity and to improve the function of the MP joints. Of the implant replacements, Swanson silicone rubber implant arthroplasty continues to be the most popular, although minimal gain in motion [8], recurrence of some degree of ulnar deformity, and fractures of implants are reported [9]. In this paper we report on our experience of Swanson silicone rubber implant arthroplasty of MP joints in RA.

Patients and Methods

From 1974 to 1983 Swanson silicone rubber implant arthroplasty was performed on 37 hands (32 patients, 26 females and 6 males) in a total of 107 MP joints (II MP 31, III MP 28, IV and V MP joints both 24 implants). The number of right hands was 27 and of left hands 10. All four MP joints were replaced in 20 hands, whereas in the other 17 hands from one to three MP joints were replaced.

The mean age of the patients at the time of the operation was 60 years (27–78) and the duration of RA and hand symptoms 16.6 and 16 years, respectively (range 4–40 years). Synovectomy of the MP joints was performed in only one hand 6 years before arthroplasty.

We examined the patients clinically in 1984. AP and lateral view radiographs of both hands were taken. In our follow-up study we recorded the following data: pinch strength, range of active extension and flexion, ulnar deviation of the fingers during active maximum extension, the minimum distance between the tip of the finger pulp and

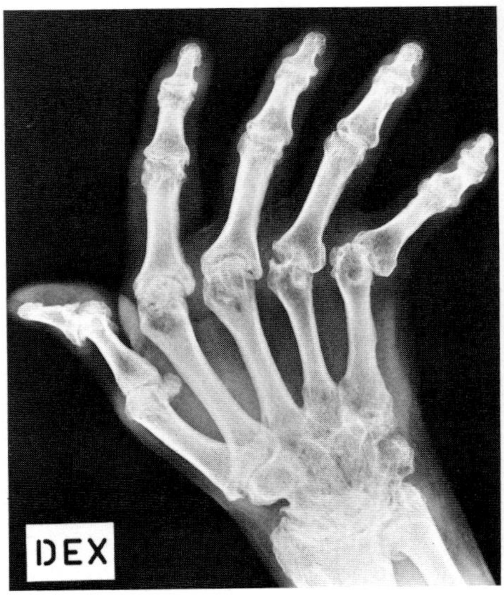

1

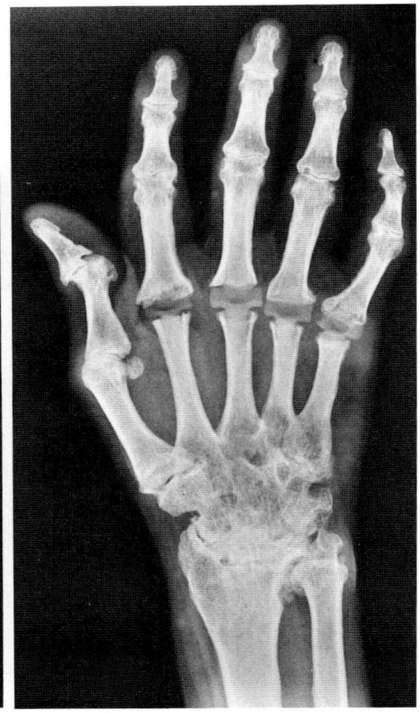

2

Fig. 1. The right hand of a 47-year-old female patient with symptoms of RA of about 30 years' duration.

Fig. 2. The same hand (as in fig. 1) after silastic rubber implant arthroplasty of the second to fifth MP joints.

the palm, relief of pain, functioning in daily activities [11], as well as the subjective cosmetic result.

From the radiographs we investigated possible dislocation of an implant or a joint, fracture of an implant or a bone, bone resorption and migration of an implant, and bone production around the stem, or junction of the hinge and stem of an implant.

Surgical Technique

We generally perform synovectomy as a first operation combined with ulnar release in cases where the alignment of the MP joint is still satisfactory, even if there is a

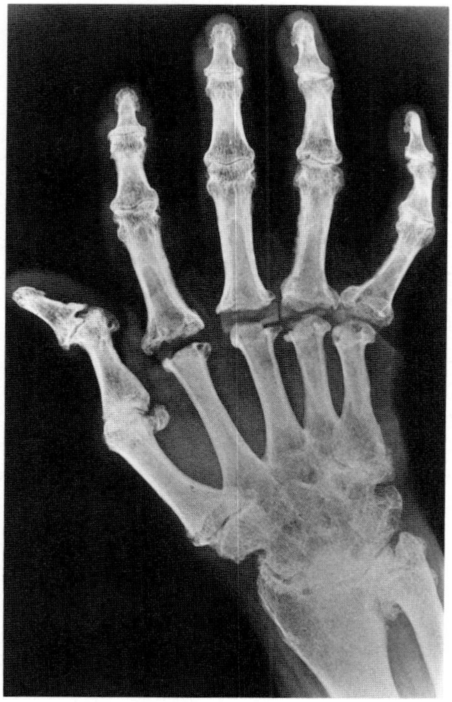

Fig. 3. The same hand (as in fig. 1, 2) 4 years later. Bone production appearing as osteophytes in the metacarpals. Increased ulnar deviation in the fourth and fifth fingers. The functioning of the MP joints is good with an active motion from zero (full extension) to 50° (index and middle fingers) and to 60° of flexion (ring and little fingers). However, the patient cannot reach the palm with the second to fourth fingers because of the stiffness of the PIP joints. The pinch against to the thumb is possible.

tendency to ulnar deviation. In the case of a flexor or extensor tendon rupture we perform reconstructions first and use dynamic splints in the aftercare, if necessary. As a first-stage operation on the hand we generally perform operations on the proximal interphalangeal joints (PIP), together with wrist operations (e.g. arthrodesis) and after that MP arthroplasty [10]. In the patients of our study no other major operations were performed – at the same time as a Swanson arthroplasty – except for stabilization or synovectomy of the joints of the thumb or of one or two PIP joints.

The replacement arthroplasty was performed through a dorsal transverse skin incision proximal to the metacarpal head. The technique described e.g. by Swanson [5, 6], and Nalebuff [7] was employed with slight modifications. Extensive capsular and intrinsic release on the ulnar side was always carried out. The extensor indicis proprius tendon was transposed to the radial side of the proximal phalanx in nearly all cases, whereas the intrinsic tendon of the third finger was in a few cases transposed to the dorsoradial extensor hood of the proximal phalanx of the fourth finger. The abductor and flexor brevis tendons of the fifth finger were cut in cases of severe ulnar drift (about 45° of ulnar deviation or more). The volar plate of the MP joint was resected in cases of flexion contracture, volar luxation or severe ulnar drift of the MP joint. The narrow medullary canals, usually in the 4th and 5th metacarpals, were enlarged by drilling so that an implant of at least size No. 4 or 5 could be inserted into these fingers. In the other fingers, implants of sizes 6, 7 or 8 were used. The radial collateral ligament was sutured to the dorsoradial edge of the metacarpal bone or to the remnants of the capsulae. No attempt to reconstruct the radial collateral ligament (e.g. with a strip of the volar plate) was made. The midposition of the extensor tendon was aimed for. Suction drainage was almost always used. Prophylactic antibiotic treatment was given for 2 days.

On the third postoperative day the compression bandage was removed and a dynamic splint with dorsoradial pull was applied, and flexion and extension of the fingers was encouraged. During the last year, in the case of a painful or unstable PIP joint, a small dorsal splint was used to stabilize the PIP joint, because stabilization of a severely damaged PIP joint (especially of the 5th finger) helps the mobilization of the MP joint [10].

During the night for the first 3 weeks a flexion bandage or a flexion cuff was often used to keep the MP and PIP joints in flexion. But recently we have preferred to use a dynamic plastic splint with the possibility of pulling the proximal phalanx into extension or flexion. The dynamic extension splint was used for about 2 months.

Results

The mean active range of motion (ROM) of all replaced MP joints was 34°. Active maximal motion of the second MP joint ranged from 0° to 70° (from full extension to maximal flexion). The respective values of the third MP joint were from 0° to 60°, of the fourth MP joint from 0° to 60° and of the fifth MP joint from 0° to 80°. The mean active extension deficit of all the replaced MP joints was 7° (range from 0° to 30°). Mean values of extension deficit and active flexion of the different fingers are shown in table I. The differences in values between the different MP joints were slight.

An active flexion of the MP joint of less than 30° was found in 20 replaced joints (5 MP II joints, 6 MP III, 4 MP IV and 5 MP V) in a total of eight hands, i.e. in 19% (20/107) of all implants. The mean follow-up time in these cases was 61.5 months, which is clearly longer than the average follow-up time for all the cases (44.5 months). Active motion of the PIP joints was spontaneously severely restricted or one or two PIP joints were arthrodesed, in six of these eight hands.

Table I. Silicone rubber implant arthroplasty of the MP joints in rheumatoid arthritis. Average active extension/flexion in degrees and ulnar deviation of the fingers at the follow-up examination

Finger No. 107	Ext./flex.	Ulnar deviation		
		Average in degrees	more than 10°	
			number	percent
II	-6/42	9	7/31	23
III	-10/40	11	9/28	32
IV	-6/42	12	7/24	29
V	-6/40	15	10/24	42
Mean	-7/41		33/107	31

Active flexion of 60° or more was found in 36 replaced MP joints (34%) at the follow-up examination.

The shortest distance between the tip of the second to fifth fingers and the palm in active maximal flexion of the fingers ranged from 0 to 50 mm (mean 13–19 mm). In 7 cases of operated index fingers (7/31, 23%) the tip of the finger touched the palm, this was present in 9 middle fingers (9/28, 32%) and in 9 ring and little fingers (9/24, 37%), respectively.

An ulnar deviation of more than 10° was measured in 33/107 fingers (31%) and deviation of more than 5° was found in 50 fingers (47%) (fig. 1–3). The mean ulnar deviation of the index finger was 9°, of the middle finger 11°, of the ring and little fingers 12° and 15°, respectively. The values of ulnar deformity in different fingers are shown in table I.

Active pinch strength of each finger with a Swanson implant (one finger at the time pressed against the thumb) was measured with a vigometer (Osco Downey, Calif.). All the patients were right-handed. The highest value of the pinch grip was that of the right index finger, 6.8 kg. Mean values are shown in table II.

Pain relief was generally good; mild pain in the replaced joint was experienced in 16% of the hands. Functioning of the fingers in daily ac-

Table II. Silicone rubber implant arthroblasty of the MP joints in rheumatoid arthritis. Active pinch strength of one finger against the thumb at the follow-up examination (mean values in kg)

	Index	Middle	Ring	Little
Right hand	4.1	2.3	1.8	1.4
Left hand	2.3	1.4	0.9	0.4

Range of values from 0 to 6.8 kg.

tivities (as a subjective assessment by the patients) was satisfactory in 31 hands (84%) and was poorly limited in the remaining six hands. The cosmetic result, according to the patients, was acceptable in 32 hands (86%). Nonacceptable disabling stiffness of the replaced MP joints, assessed by the patients, was reported in only 11% (12/107 implants). None of the patients developed a proved deep bacterial infection, and there were no cases of necrosis of the skin requiring surgical procedures or prolonged antibiotic treatment.

Radiological Findings

Confirmed fracture of the hinge of an implant was found in four implants (4%). The fracture was confirmed if a marked derotation of the stems or marked dislocation or subluxation of the joint was found. Two implant fractures were operatively confirmed and new implants were inserted. The fracture of an implant was suspected if the joint was not displaced but the proximal or distal stem of an implant was clearly rotated and the finger deviated ulnarly. This suspicion was found in 10% of implants (table III).

Bone overgrowth was found in only 9% of cases but bone resorption was present, in a total of 26 cases (24%), around the hinge of an implant or around the distal stem (4 cases). Bone resorption was mostly found in the index finger (10 cases). None of the implants was displaced out of the bone. Migration of an implant together with bone resorption was clearly observed in 25 cases (23%). It was found in the index finger in 9 cases, in the middle finger in 6, and in the ring and little fingers in 5 cases each. Two minor fractures of the proximal phalanx of

Table III. Silicone rubber implant arthroblasty of the MP joints in rheumatoid arthritis. Radiological findings at the follow-up examination

	Number	Percent
Bone resorption around an implant	26/107	24
Migration of an implant	25/107	23
Bone overgrowth around the hinge	10/107	9
Confirmed fracture of an implant	4/107	4
Probable fracture of an implant	11/107	10
Surgical complication: fracture of bone (1 phalanx, 1 MC)	2/107	2

the index finger and the distal edge of the second metacarpal bone appeared as a surgical complication and they healed without troubles.

Discussion

The mean active ROM of the replaced joints (Swanson implants) has been reported to be very close to 40° [8, 9, 12, 13]. In our report the mean active ROM was 34° (from -7° to 41°). The gain of the mean active ROM over the preoperative values was 5° according to Mannerfelt and Andersson [8] and 17° according to Blair et al. [9]. Mean ROM did not differ much between the second and other replaced MP joints [8], as we also found. Swanson [6] reported much better ROM values, of 61.5° (from -2.5° to 64°) and 53° (from -4° to 57°) in a follow-up of from 6 months to 5 years after surgery. However, these values were recorded as a passive ROM. In our study the most severe pathology was present preoperatively in replaced MP joints with a long history of rheumatoid disease. This may be one reason for the stiffness of the replaced joints. Another reason may be the lack of passive flexion therapy - flexion cuffs or dynamic splints. Nowadays we use these methods in physical aftercare.

According to Blair et al. [9] a flexion of 40° should be achieved with silicone rubber implants, if there are no postoperative complications. This degree of flexion allows the touching of the palm with the tip of the finger, if the function of the PIP joint is normal or nearly normal. This is not possible in many rheumatoid hands.

The frequency of an ulnar deviation deformity of 30° or more in the earlier reports varies from less than 1 to 9.5% of cases and the recurrence frequency from 9.7% [13] to 43% [9]. In our patients an ulnar deviation of over 30° was found in 9/107 fingers but of more than 10° in 31% of cases. This was more advanced in the fifth finger. Much care should be given to the releasing of the ulnar side soft tissues and to the use of the maximum size of implant. We found that no implant had perforated the cortex but osteolytic areas and migration of an implant were common (in 24% of the cases) especially around the hinge of an implant.

Fractures were found in only 4 implants but were suspected in 11 more implants. On a usual radiograph – without a stress examination – fracture of an implant may be very difficult to see. Therefore, the frequency of fractures is probably higher than 4%. None of the damaged implants caused painful synovitis of the joint and a possible reoperation was indicated only in the case of a severe deformity or a poor function of a finger. This finding, as well as the rareness of deep infection, are in accordance with the earlier reports. The reported frequency of fracture of an implant is a little higher than in our study –26.2% [13] and 21% [9], probably because the older types of implant were made of weaker material. Mannerfelt and Andersson [8] reported only four fractures in 144 implants. Blair et al. [9] also found bone resorption around an implant in many cases, as we did, and in time this may lead to decreased functioning of an implant or even to fractures and dislocation of a joint. In such a case the possibility of rearthroplasty resulting in satisfactory functioning is diminished.

In conclusion we found, despite of some deterioration of the results in cases of a long-term follow-up, that this method in prosthetic replacement of the MP joints in RA is useful. Special regard should be given to good alignment of the wrist and satisfactory function or stability of the PIP joints before the MP implant arthroplasty. The successful balancing of dynamic forces by soft tissue release and a longlasting physiotherapy of the hand are important.

Summary

We evaluated Swanson's silicone rubber implant arthroplasty of the metacarpophalangeal joint by retrospective analysis in 32 rheumatoid patients (37 hands). One hundred and seven implants were followed up for an average of 44.5 (12–120) months.

The active motion of the metacarpophalangeal joint averaged 34°, the mean extension deficit being 7° and the mean flexion 41°. Ulnar deviation recurred to more than 10° in 33/107 fingers (31%). Fracture of the spacer was confirmed in four joints (4%). One fracture of the proximal phalanx and one of the metacarpal bone had occurred. Bone resorption around the stem or a hinge and migration of the implant was found in 26 (24%) fingers. Patient satisfaction was high; 27 patients experienced significant pain relief, the functioning of 31 hands (84%) was improved and 28 patients (32 hands) thought that the cosmetic appearance of the hand was improved.

References

1 Riordan, D.C.; Fowler, S.B.: Surgical treatment of rheumatoid deformities of the hand. J. Bone Jt Surg. *40:* 1431–1432 (1958).

2 Straub, L.R.: The rheumatoid hand. Clin. Orthop. *15:* 127–139 (1959).

3 Vainio, K.J.: The rheumatoid hand; in Milch, Surgery of arthritis, pp. 130–158 (Williams & Wilkins, Baltimore 1964).

4 Flatt, A.E.: The care of the rheumatoid hand (Mosby, St. Louis 1963).

5 Swanson, A.B.: Silicone rubber implants for replacement of arthritic or destroyed joints in the hand. Surg. Clins N. Am. *48:* 1113–1127 (1968).

6 Swanson, A.B.: Flexible implant arthroplasty for arthritic finger joints. Rationale, technique and results of treatment. J. Bone Jt Surg. *54:* 435–455 (1972).

7 Nalebuff, E.A.: Metacarpophalangeal surgery in rheumatoid arthritis. Surg. Clins N. Am. *49:* 823–832 (1969).

8 Mannerfelt, L.; Andersson, K.: Silastic arthroplasty of the metacarpophalangeal joints in rheumatoid arthritis. Long-term results. J. Bone Jt Surg. *57:* 484–489 (1975).

9 Blair, W.F.; Shurr, D.G.; Buckwalter, J.A.: Metacarpophalangeal joint implant arthroplasty with a Silastic spacer. J. Bone Jt Surg. *66:* 365–370 (1984).

10 Nalebuff, E.A.: The rheumatoid hand. Reflections on metacarpophalangeal arthroplasty. Clin. Orthop. *182:* 150–159 (1984).

11 Swanson, A.B.: Flexible implant resection arthroplasty in the hand and extremities, pp. 92–118 (Mosby, St. Louis 1973).

12 Gschwend, N.; Zimmermann, J.: Analyse von 200 MCP-Arthroplastiken. Handchirurgie *6:* 7–14 (1974).

13 Beckenbaugh, R.D.; Dobyns, J.H.; Linscheid, R.L.; Bryan, R.S.: Review and analysis of silicone-rubber metacarpophalangeal implants. J. Bone Jt Surg. *58:* 483–487 (1976).

Dr. Veijo Vahvanen, The Orthopaedic Hospital of the Invalid Foundation,
Tenholantie 10, SF-00280 Helsinki 28 (Finland)

Rheumatology, vol. 11, pp. 80–91 (Karger, Basel 1987)

Assessment of the Functional Gain of Various Operations in the Complex Hand

N. Gschwend

Klinik Wilhelm Schulthess, Zürich, Schweiz

Introduction

Everybody agrees that the real art in dealing with the operative treatment of rheumatoid arthritis (RA) consists in setting up a therapeutic plan with priorities. Good operative technique is a prerequisite. Deformity per se is not an indication for operation. We do not operate X-rays, but patients who are suffering and asking for pain relief or functional improvement when conservative methods have failed. In this view we should try more to evaluate our operation, answering the question whether we really improve daily functions and whether this improvement is a lasting one. As an example let us take the arthroplasty of the MP joint. There is no doubt that cosmetics has improved in almost all cases to a considerable extent. In most cases we gain extension, but we might lose flexion. We therefore should test complex functions of daily living and analyze whether the operation allows the patient to do things which he was not able to do before surgery. Such

Table I. Patients assessment in MCP arthroplasty: Swanson design (1974–82)

Functional improvement		
Remarkable improvement	40%	
Slight improvement	25%	
None	20%	35%
Worse	15%	

Self-care	Activities	100 %	75 %	50 %	25 %	0 %	Functional handicap	Measures envisaged
Eating, %	with knife/fork							
	with spoon							
	drinking with cup							
	drinking with glass							
Hygiene, %	shower/bath							
	washing							
	drying							
	intimate care/WC							
	hair-dressing							
	cleaning of teeth							
	shaving/make up							
Dressing, %	coat							
	jumper/dress							
	jacket/shirt							
	underwear/bra							
	stockings/socks							
	lacing of shoes							
	buttons							
	zip-fastener							
Legend, %	100						*without* difficulty (not troublesome, without any restriction)	
	75						*with* difficulty (troublesome, i.e. slowed by pain or slightly restrictive movement)	
	50						with *auxiliary devices* (only with latter, adaptation or special tool)	
	25						with *help by other person* (with some contribution by patient)	
	0						*not* possible (completely dependent)	

Fig. 1. Special sheets with test questions for self-care.

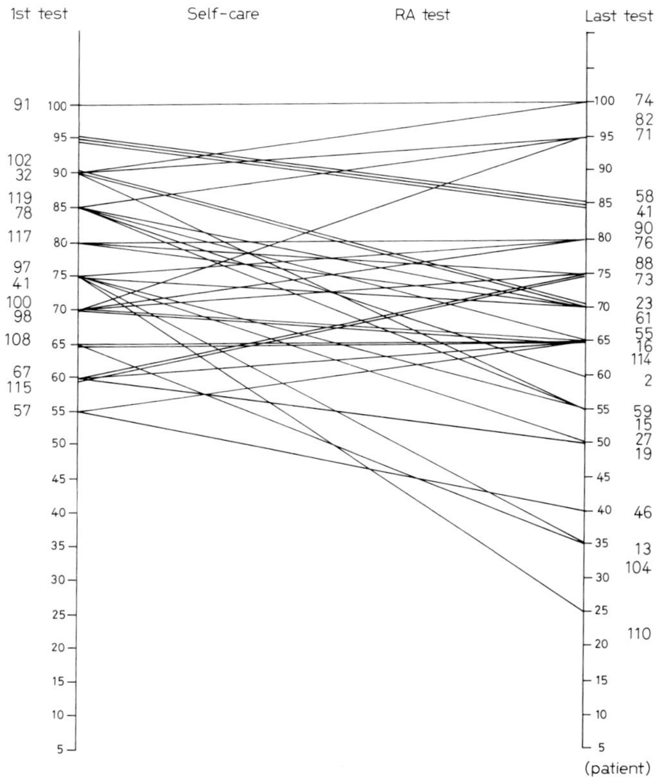

Fig. 2, 3. Test curves of various cases in which the first test and the last test were 5–10 years apart: they reflect more the natural course of the disease with gradually increasing invalidity.

considerations came up to our mind by analyzing a consecutive series of 207 joints, where the second generation of Swanson Silastic prostheses, made of high performance silastomer, has been used. The average follow-up was 56 months, a minimum of 12 months was required, the maximum reached 114 months. Whereas pain relief was obtained in a very high proportion of the operated cases, functional improvement in more than one third of the cases was not achieved (table I). Only 40% showed a remarkable improvement of complex function. On

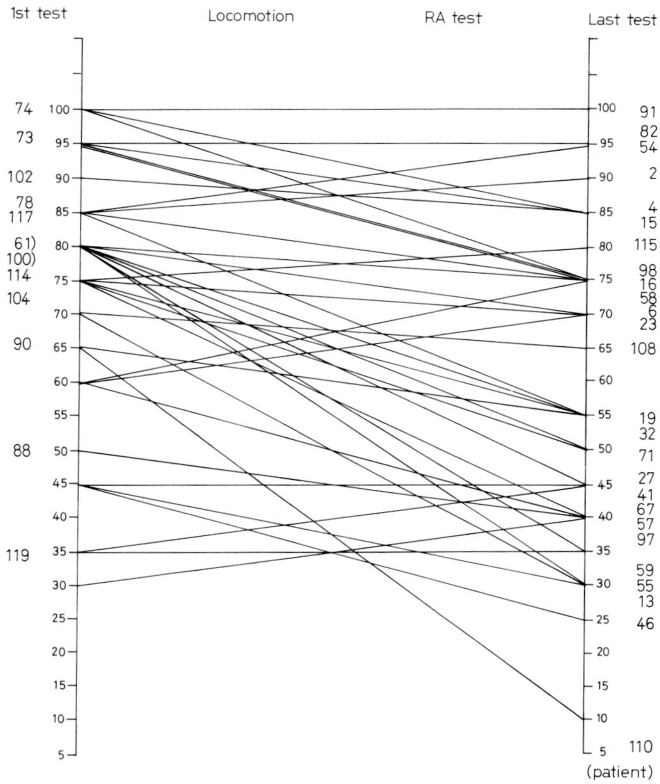

Fig. 3. For legend see opposite side.

the other hand it was amazing to see that 92% of the patients declared themselves very satisfied, which may be due particularly to the high percentage of pain relief and cosmetical improvement. The reason why many of these hands do not provide the patient with a functional improvement was certainly due to a lack of finger flexion. Only one third of all the patients was able to make a fist. Lack of active extension of more than 30° was noted in 20% of the patients. The range of active motion was in fact slightly diminished.

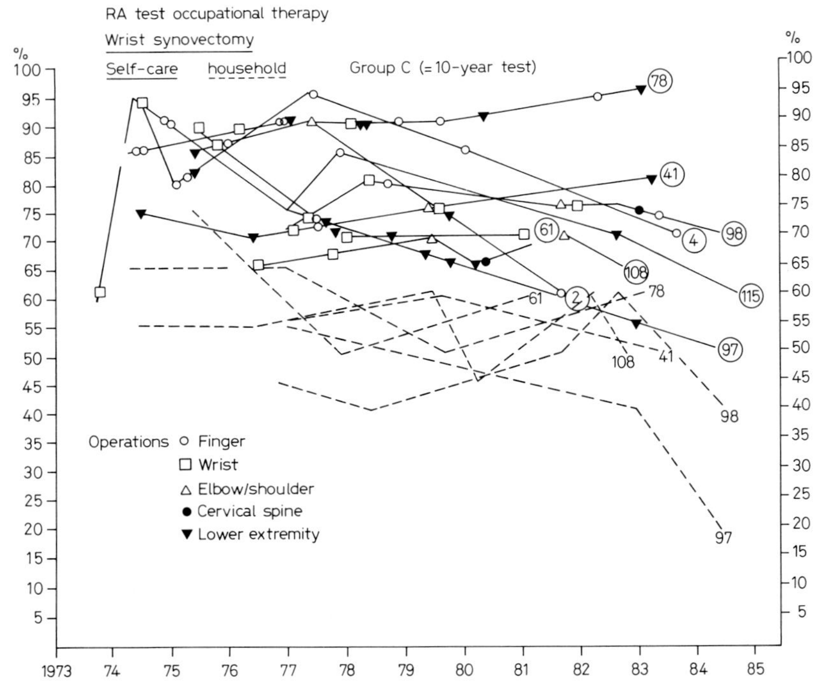
RA test occupational therapy
Wrist synovectomy
Self-care
household
Group C (=10-year test)
%
Operations ○ Finger
□ Wrist
△ Elbow/shoulder
● Cervical spine
▼ Lower extremity
1973 74 75 76 77 78 79 80 81 82 83 84 85

4

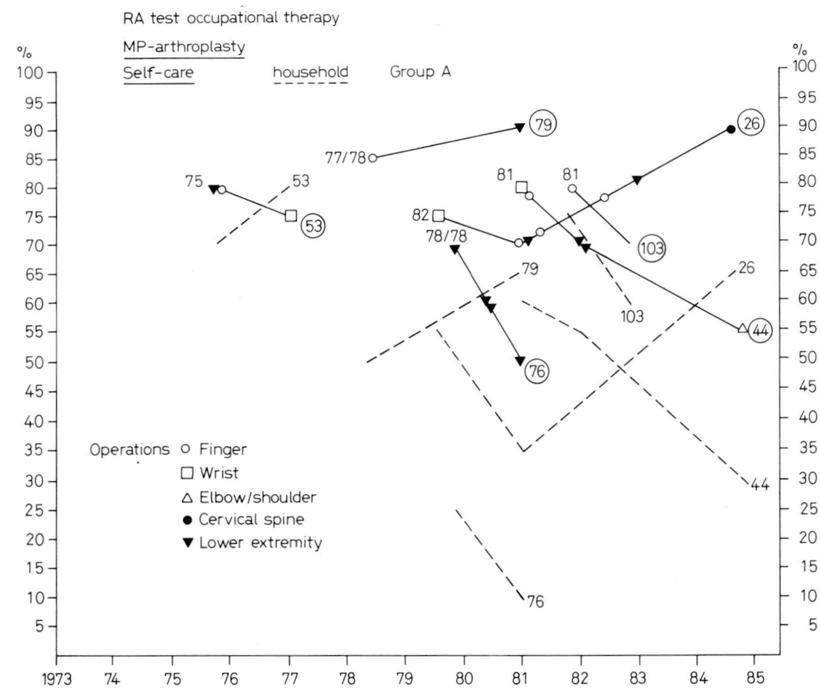
RA test occupational therapy
MP-arthroplasty
Self-care
household
Group A
%
Operations ○ Finger
□ Wrist
△ Elbow/shoulder
● Cervical spine
▼ Lower extremity
1973 74 75 76 77 78 79 80 81 82 83 84 85

5

K.J. 1922 Positive result

1982 MP arthroplasty 2–5 right

1984 Fist: lack of full flexion 1 cm
Deformity corrected

1984 Arthroplasty wrist left

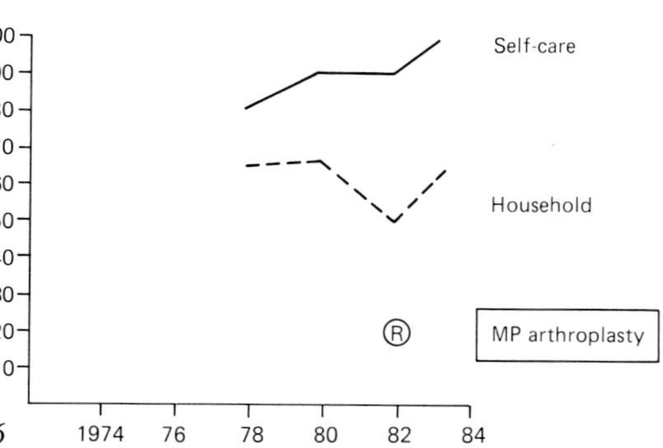

6

M.M. 1925 negative result

1975 Arthroplasty MP 2–5 left

1976 Arthroplasty MP 2–5 right
Synovectomy PIP 3 left
Arthrodesis IP 1 left
Caput ulnae resection left

Increasing difficulty with *left shoulder* and *right thumb*

Hand and finger function good, patient satisfied

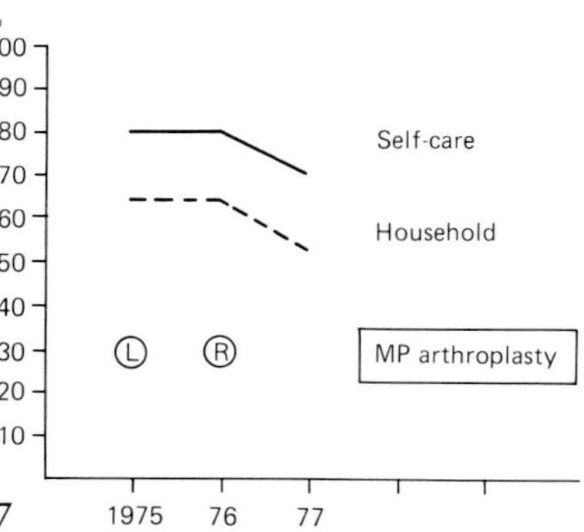

7

O.A. 1929 negative result

1974 Arthroplasty MP 2–5 right
Synovectomy PIP 2 left
After 6 months arthroplasty MP 2–5 left
After 10 months extensor tenosynovectomy right
Swan-neck 3 and 4 soft tissue procedure

Severe thumb deformity (90/90) requiring arthrodesis 1985

1980 Arthroplasty knee joint R + l

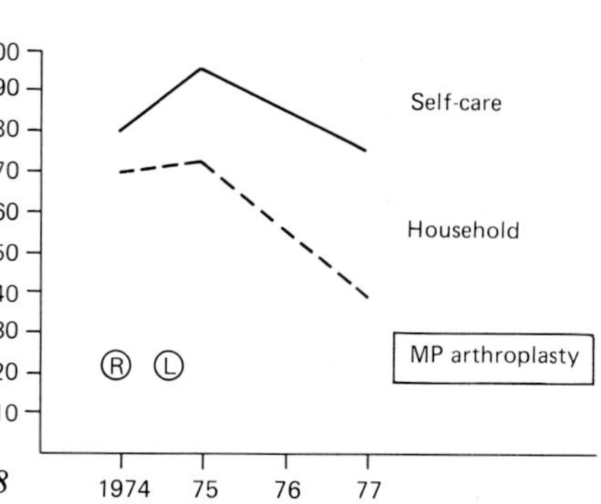

8

S.G. 1931 negative result

1975 Arthroplasty MP 2–5 right
Hand funtion not improved

1976 Pain and reduced ROM *right shoulder*

1977 Elbow revision for arthroplasty

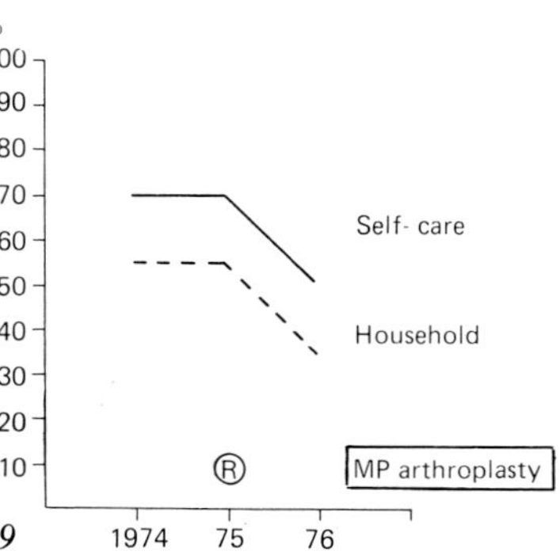

9

Fig. 6–11. Functional test curves of individual cases having undergone various operations at the wrist and/or finger level.

Fig. 4, 5. The first and last test are only 1–3 years apart. This allows us a more reliable appraisal of the value of operated procedures done in this period.

B.M. 1943 positive result

1979 Wrist arthroplasty left + resection ulnar head

1981 Arthroplasty MP 2–5 right
Arthrodesis MP 1 right

1982 Arthrodesis MP 1 left
MP 2–5 arthroplasty left

Fist: full flexion both hands

Other operation forefoot
C 1–2 fusion

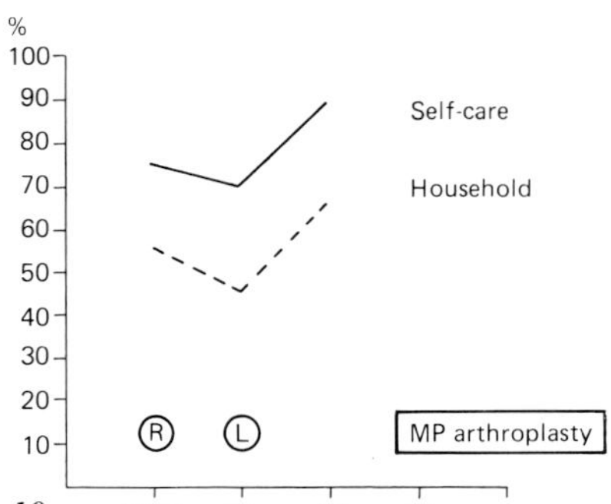

10

G.H. 1935 negative result

1981 Swanson arthroplasty right wrist
Swanson MP arthroplasty 2–5 right hand

1982 Poor flexion MP and PIP (60–80°)
Instability right thumb
Fist: lack of full flexion preop. 0 cm
postop. 4 cm

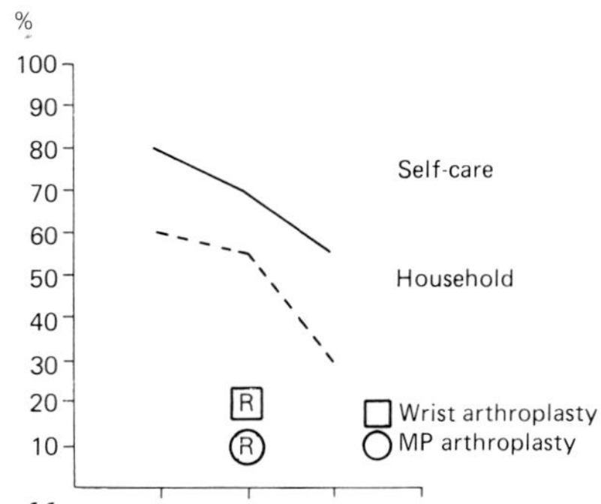

11

Fig. 10, 11. For legend see p. 85.

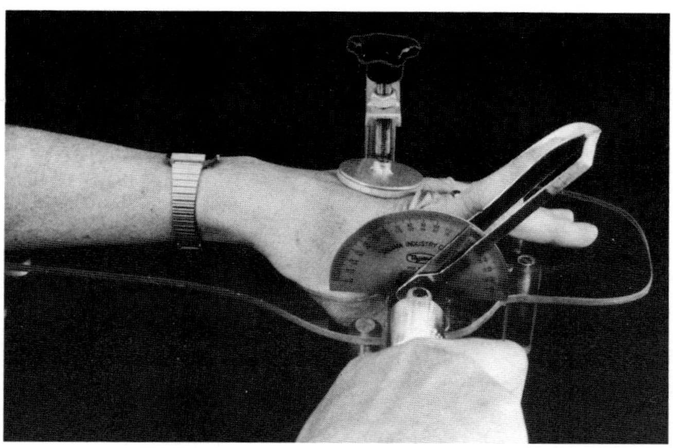

Fig. 12. Constitutional joint laxity: the hyperextension test machine.

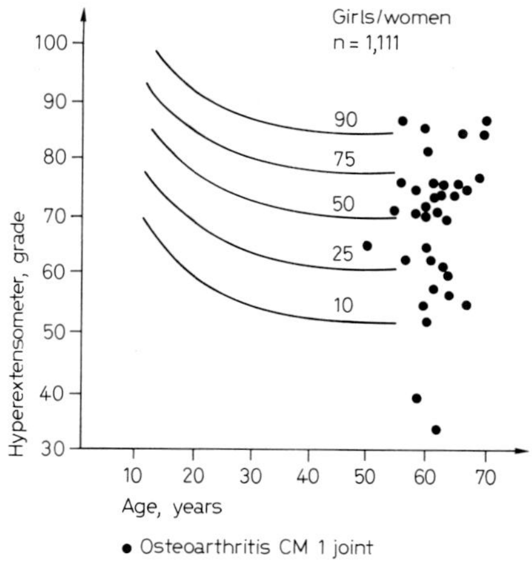

Fig. 13. The importance of constitutional joint laxity in osteoarthritis of the CM 1 joint: the majority had values above average hyperextension.

Our Functional Testing System

In order to evaluate surgery from a more functional point of view, we have been using special sheets with test questions for self-care (fig. 1), household, locomotion and profession for more than 10 years. In addition to these questions, practical tests have been executed. For the various functions in daily living, we estimated the functional impairment in percentages. This means that being able to do a given function without difficulties was allotted 100%. If some difficulties were noted: 75%. If the function could only be executed by the use of rheuma aids: 50%; if foreign help of another person was needed: 25%; to a complete loss of a given function 0% was allocated. The summation of all the percentages was noted and the test repeated in various intervals. 480 tests in 148 RA patients, of which 122 were female, were analyzed. In this present study we were particularly interested in comparing the tests for self-care and household before and after operations at wrists and fingers. If the interval between the first and the last test is long, i.e. more than 5 years, then the natural course of this type of RA is reflected. It will be difficult to estimate the value of a given operation in such a case as many non-operated joints may have deteriorated in the meantime. For estimating the value of an operation, we therefore

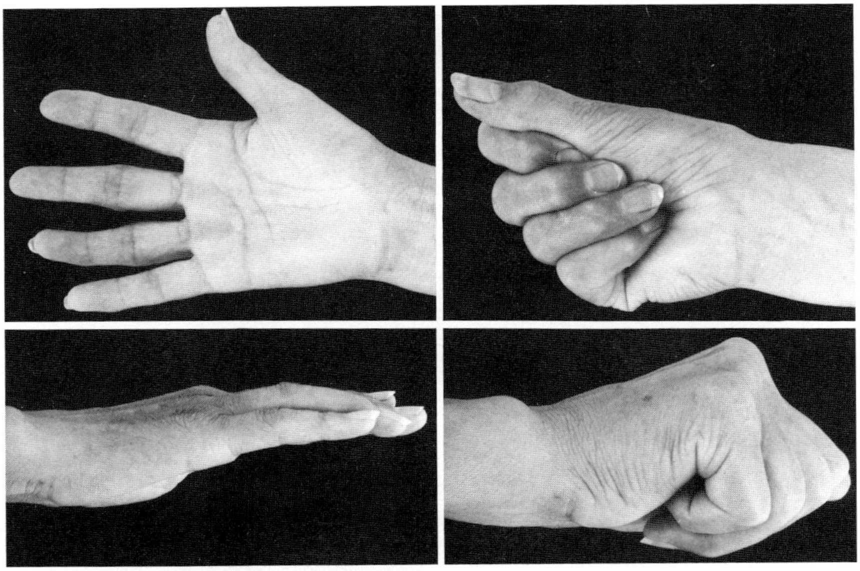

14

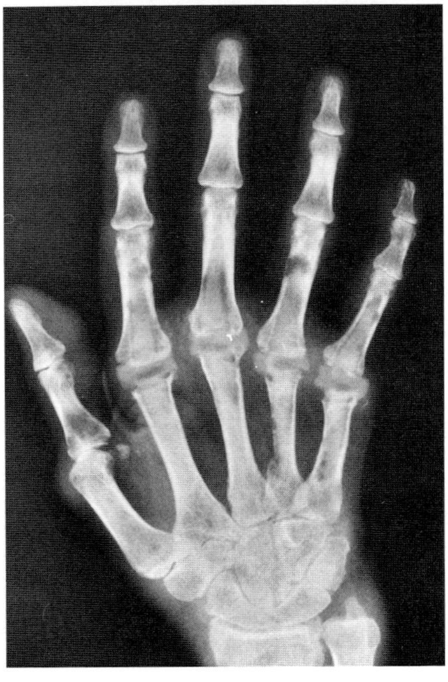

15

Fig. 14, 15. Due to a constitutionally increased joint laxity, Silastic arthroplasty of MP II–V resulted in an excellent mobility. The disadvantage: bone resorption due to pistoning, wear and foreign body reaction.

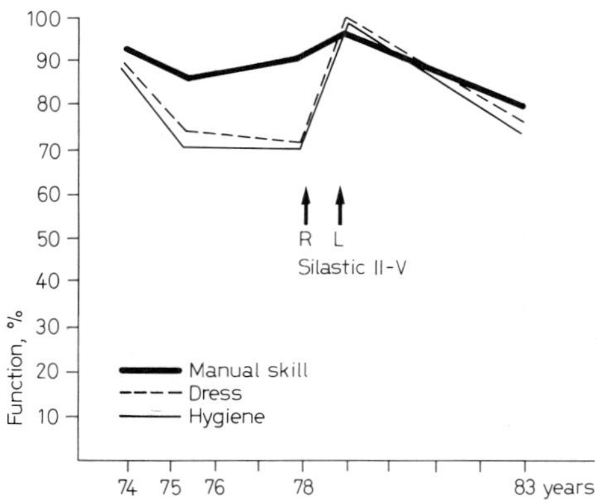

Fig. 16. Test curves of a lady who underwent MP arthroplasty on the right hand with great profit. The deterioration of function after the same procedure on the left hand occurred because of an increasing disability of the left shoulder.

choose cases in which the first test and the last one were only 1–3 years apart. Figures 2 and 3 show the curves of various cases in which the first test and the last one were 5–10 years apart. We see that in most cases, according to the progressive nature of the disease, invalidity increased, or in other words, the degree of independence in self-care and locomotion decreased percentagewise. On the other hand in figures 4 and 5, where the interval is relatively short, we see many cases in which a deterioration can be detected, but on the other hand there are also cases in which a clear-cut improvement can be seen.

Results

The analysis of individual cases gives us a picture which is shown in the figures 6–11. Summarizing these individual cases, we see that in many cases metacarpophalangeal (MP) arthroplasty as a typical example may improve considerably the complex function of self-care, provided a good mobility is obtained and especially that the function of thumb and proximal interphalangeal (PIP) joints is at least acceptable. On the other hand, arthroplasty of the MP joint will not prevent a further deterioration if the elbow or shoulder joint is mainly or increasingly affected. Some of the negative results prove the importance of a

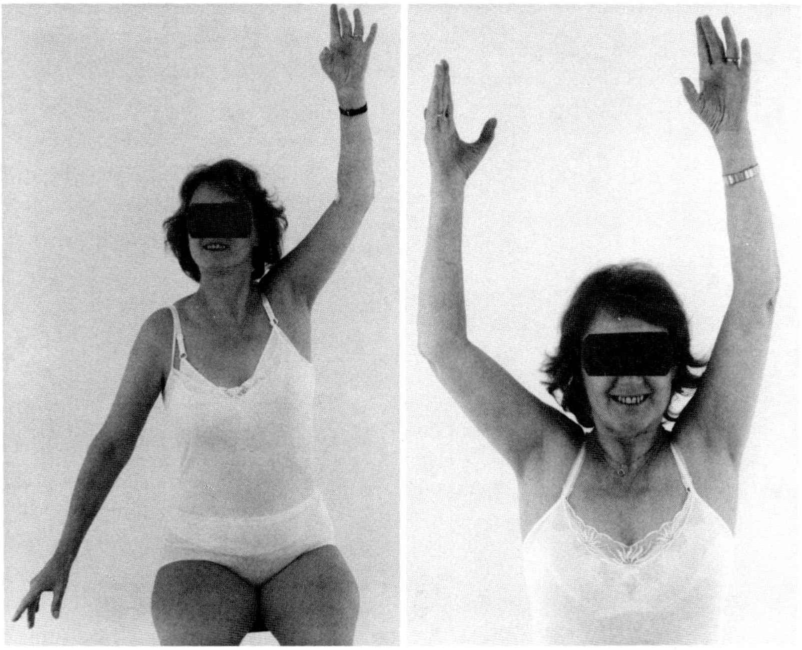

Fig. 17. After shoulder arthroplasty the function in daily living improved considerably.

careful preoperative evaluation of all individual joints in order to find out the main cause of a given handicap. Only by doing this shall we be able to avoid unnecessary operations or even a deterioration by our surgical efforts.

When mobility of the joints, e.g. after MP arthroplasties, is concerned, it not only depends on the surgical skill and after treatment, but perhaps even more on the individual constitutional joint laxity. Having done several thousand hyperextension tests (fig. 12) of the MP 2 of the left hand in normal individuals and in patients with different diseases, we were able to produce curves for the various ages and the two sexes. Doing the same hyperextension test on the MP II joint of the left hand in cases with osteoarthritis of the carpometacarpal joint 1, we were able to demonstrate that most patients had an above-average laxity of ligaments (fig. 13). This proves the validity of the assumption that joint laxity is one of the important pathogenetic factors in this disease.

On the other hand, it also explains why it is often difficult to stabilize an implant after surgery, and why subluxation and even dislocation are to be found relatively frequently. Unfortunately, these tests can practically never be applied in RA because of an involvement of the MP II joint in most cases. It would give us the possibility to predict the mobility before surgery and to restrict indications for 'stiff-types' to only those cases, where the PIP joints are normal and where the thumb may be able to compensate for a reduced MP mobility. That joint laxity is not only advantageous is shown in figures 14 and 15, where after MP arthroplasty an excellent mobility has been obtained, but where this excessive mobility led to an early bone resorption by a pistoning effect of the silastic implant, and therefore increased wear and foreign body reaction. Figure 16 shows the value of the presented testing method in a lady who obviously profited by an MP arthroplasty of the right hand, but whose left hand deteriorated in function after the operation. The reason was not the operation but the fact that we overlooked that the patient was mainly handicapped by her right shoulder. Shoulder arthroplasty immediately improved the complex function considerably (fig. 17). From a functional point of view, the operation of the MP of the left hand could have been dispensed with.

Summarizing, we would like to say that it will be our duty in the future to look at our surgical activity more from a point of view of complex functions, keeping in mind that the hand and finger are only single elements in a functional chain which has to be looked at as a whole.

Prof. Dr. Norbert Gschwend, Klinik Wilhelm Schulthess, Neumünsterallee 3, CH-8008 Zürich (Schweiz)

Rheumatology, vol. 11, pp. 92–96 (Karger, Basel 1987)

The Complex Hand – Round Table Discussion

W.A. Souter, Y. Allieu, N. Gschwend, S. Jakubowski, P. Raunio, J. Teigland

At the start of the discussion, the Chairman invited two notes of caution from Prof. Allieu whose studies on function after multiple hand surgery had shown that the improvement in function was inversely proportional to the number of operations. In other words, it appeared that if the problem was too complex, surgery might effect very little, unless the patient's disability was very carefully analysed and the surgical management restricted to one or two key operations designed to restore specific aspects of function. A massive surgical onslaught was all too liable to jeopardise the residual function of the grossly deformed hand. The second point he wished to make was that operations which were normally very successful might not be so in the rheumatoid hand because of pre-existing muscle imbalance.

Dr. Bosch (Netherlands) agreed with this and stated that it was their impression that too much surgery resulted in irreversible stiffness of the hand. He consequently deprecated any major trend towards carrying out multiple operations on the hand at one sitting.

Mr. Porter (UK) requested the panel's view on fusion of the distal interphalangeal (DIP) joints in the presence of marked erosions and also on the management of mutilans deformities. It was generally agreed that the use of bone grafts was essential if fusion was to be achieved. Silastic implants could also be helpful in maintaining length and offering at least for a time some stability of fulcra.

Dr. Bosch also asked if it was possible to forecast the development of different patterns of hand deformity, but the panel felt that this was not so.

Comments on the value of alternative procedures to the use of silastic spacers at the metacarpophalangeal (MCP) joints were requested from the floor. It was the panel's view that Vainio's arthroplasty in highly skilled hands was a valuable procedure but the Tupper arthroplasty was equally effective and perhaps easier to perform.

Dr. König (FRG) asked about resection of the ulnar head in the course of dorsal wrist surgery - when was it indicated and should it be preserved, if its articular cartilage was undamaged? The panel conceded that there might be theoretical grounds for preserving it in a very few cases. Nevertheless in practice the radio-ulnar joint was usually significantly involved and the head of the ulna often unstable because of destruction of the triangular articular disc. It was generally felt that while one might well regret leaving it, if radio-ulnar involvement occured later, one very seldom had any regrets regarding its removal.

The question of poor results with regard to movement after synovectomy and MCP joint arthroplasty in psoriatic arthropathy was raised. The panel agreed that this was a problem and expressed the view that this was most likely to be due to an enhanced tendency to form scar tissue.

Dr. Jaffe (South Africa) sought the panel's views on rupture of the extensors to the little, ring and long fingers and on rupture of both flexors to a single digit. With regard to the latter, it was felt that if a sublimis tendon was available in the neighbouring digit, it should be transposed to the distal stump of the flexor digitorum profundus in the affected finger. Where the rupture had occurred in 'no man's land', the temporary use of a silastic rod followed later by tendon grafting appeared to be the method of choice. With regard to multiple ruptures of extensor tendons, it was felt that end-to-side suture of adjacent tendons became impracticable and transposition of the extensor indicis proprius offered the best chance of a good functional result.

The second part of the panel discussion was devoted to a consideration of the points made earlier in the day by Dr. Mannerfelt regarding the priorities of surgery in the complex rheumatoid hand. Some divergence of opinion was expressed on the following points.

Dominant before Non-Dominant

Here it was felt no absolute rule could be laid down. If there was no doubt either in the patient's or surgeon's minds as to the need for surgery, the dominant hand should probably be dealt with first. If, however, there was some doubt as to how much functional gain would be achieved, the panel felt there was a place for starting with the non-dominant hand so that the patient could then assess exactly how much or little had been gained with regard to function, and thus make an informed decision as to whether surgery on the dominant hand was likely to be worthwhile.

Button-Hole Deformity before MCP Arthroplasty

While Dr. Mannerfelt's point regarding the deleterious influence of persisting hyperextension of the MCP joint on the flexion likely to be achieved after MCP arthroplasty was well taken, several members of the panel felt that consideration also had to be given to the possibility that in the event of the postoperative movement at the MCP joints proving to be disappointing, the patient would perforce have to rely on the excellent proximal interphalangeal (PIP) joint flexion usually present in boutonnière lesions for satisfactory grasp and thus it could be argued that it was unwise to jeopardise this safeguard by preliminary surgery at PIP joint level, since stiffness at both joints would be disastrous for function.

MCP Arthroplasty before Correction of Swan-Neck Deformities

There was general agreement that the MCP joints should be dealt with first, as the former surgery might render a formal attack on the swan-neck deformities unnecessary. If, however, PIP joint arthroplasty were being contemplated as part of the surgical programme for the swan-neck correction, a simultaneous attack might be required in view of the difficulty of fitting 2 silastic stems into the medullary cavity of the proximal phalanx. In order to achieve a satisfactory fit, shortening of the stems might be required. More frequently MCP arthroplasty had to be combined with PIP joint arthrodesis.

MCP Joint Reconstruction before Extensor Tendon Repair

There was frank disagreement with this proposal by a majority of the panel, who preferred to have fully functioning extrinsic muscles before MCP reconstruction was attempted. It was conceded however that an exception to this might well have to be made in the presence of severe MCP flexion deformities.

Flexor Tendon Surgery before Extensor

This point of view also was not generally accepted as it was felt that flexor tendon surgery was too formidable a hurdle to present to the patient at the outset of treatment.

Flexor Tendon Surgery before MCP Reconstruction

This approach met with general agreement but only in the context of the extensors having already been dealt with. Dr. M. Clayton (USA) from the floor expressed the view that if the passive flexion was greater than the active, the flexor tendons should be done first. When, however, severe flexion deformities of the MCP joints were present or where there was a marked tendency to volar subluxation of these joints, the reconstruction of the MCP joints should take precedence.

Fingers before Thumb

There was a surprising amount of disagreement on this point. Some of the panel felt that surgery to the thumb, especially at the MCP joint, was such a 'winner' that it could well offer a very satisfactory starting point for a programme of reconstructive surgery. Other members of the panel believed equally strongly that the thumb should be left until the end of a surgical programme so that it could be positioned optimally at the final stage of treatment with reference to the alignment of the reconstructed fingers.

The panel emphasized that all these suggestions could only be regarded as guidelines. Any programme of surgery had to be tailored to the individual patient, the particular pattern of joint involvement with which he or she presented and his or her individual requirements.

In winding up the discussion, the Chairman stressed that Dr. Mannerfelt's message – 'Complex patient – complex disease – complex hand' – could not be overemphasised. Our reconstructive techniques were simply not sophisticated enough to cope with such a complex and finely balanced mechanism as the human hand. Real success must await the refinement of our surgical techniques to a point at which they could be exhibited with confidence at a much earlier stage of the disease while the architectural integration of the hand was still relatively intact.

W.A. Souter, FRCSE, Princess Margaret Rose Orthopaedic Hospital,
Fairmilehead, Edinbourgh, EH 107ED (England)

Rheumatology, vol. 11, pp. 97–99 (Karger, Basel 1987)

The Mutual Interplay between Forefoot and Hindfoot Affections and Deformities in RA

K. Tillmann

Orthopädische Abteilung der Rheumaklinik Bad Bramstedt GmbH,
Bad Bramstedt, FRG

According to Vahvanen [1969] pes planovalgus is by far the most frequent rheumatoid hindfoot deformity. This can be due to a more pronounced affection of the talofibular or of the fibular part of the talocrural joint. Another reason can be the widening of the mortise by instability of the distal tibiofibular joint. All these affections of the ankle joint itself are rather exceptional causes of the valgus deformity of the rheumatoid hindfoot compared to the much more frequent affections of the tarsal joints. These deformities can cause pain by pressure and secondary osteoarthrosis between the fibular malleolus and the lateral side of the calcaneus. As Kirkup [1974] has demonstrated, the pressure can even cause a stress fracture of the distal tibial diaphysis. Tarsal joint affections can cause a complete loss of the longitudinal arch and excessive forefoot abduction, which even can lead to a kind of zigzag deformity with varus position of the toes in an extreme case.

According to Vainio [1956] the talonavicular joint is the most frequently affected single tarsal joint. Additionally we found that another region with a very high rate of affections are the lateral tarsometatarsal joints [Tillmann, 1979].

As Vainio [1956] has demonstrated, the break in the tibial longitudinal arch preferably is seen distal of the mainly affected talonavicular joint. He thinks that the cuneonavicular joint has less stability compared to the talonavicular joint. In our own opinion supporting osteophytes on the dorsal side of the talonavicular joint may also prevent the break of the longitudinal arch at that place. The break in this joint itself is rather rare and maybe due to a very rapidly occurring destruction.

The shortening of the longitudinal arch seems to lead very often to an elevation of the first metatarsal bone. Another reason for this elevation can be the simultaneous or isolated destruction of the metatarsophalangeal joint of the big toe, which can be early affected. Destructions of this joint are very common and rather typical. In all these respects we could establish [Tillmann, 1979] the findings of Vainio [1956].

We think that the interplay between painful alterations of the joints of the so-called medial column [Dwyer, 1959; Evans, 1975] in the region of the hindfoot and forefoot are the key for the understanding of the typical and most frequent deformities of the rheumatoid foot. Both of them, either occurring as single affection and even more when acting together, can cause an elevation of the first metatarsal bone. The result is a flattening of the longitudinal arch and a supination of the forefoot. If this becomes fixed, the hindfoot may be pressed into a valgus position [Hohmann, 1948], when – due to the course of the disease – inflammation and pain decrease and the patient regains the ability of plantigrad walking on the forefoot. At the same time the so-called medial column, lengthened by flattening, will cause a forefoot abduction, which is favoured by the frequent destructions in the lateral tarsometatarsal joints [Tillmann, 1979].

A flattening of the longitudinal arch, supination of the first metatarsal and forefoot abduction will be the origin of the valgus deformity of the first to fourth toe. In contrast the fifth metatarsal by flattening of the transverse arch comes into a prone position. The forefoot abduction causes a relaxation of the abductor minimi muscle. This and the missing of a short extensor tendon, which favours the fibular deviation of the first four toes, leads to a varus-position of the little toe.

These reasons for toe deformity are valid not only for rheumatoid patients, but also for patients with a pronounced flatfoot and splayfoot. Moreover in rheumatoid patients simultaneous inflammation of the bursae outside and the synovitis of the joint inside as 'inflammatory tongs' may cause a more or less pronounced destruction of the abductor tendon of the big toe. Inflammatory cysts on the tibial side of the base of the first phalanx of the great toe may additionally weaken its origin. A complete dislocation of the abductor tendon to plantar as well as a rupture of this tendon allows a complete fibular luxation of the base of the proximal phalanx of the big toe.

In a similar way the 'inflammatory tongs' cause weakening and very often a rupture of the plantar fibrocatilago of the neighboured joints. The consequence is a hyperextension of the other four metatarsophalangeal joints and finally a dorsal subluxation of the bases of their proximal phalanges. These deformities become completely irreversible by an interdigital dislocation of the flexors tendons, which occur generally in these pronounced deformities.

The valgus deformity can protect the likewise frequently affected interphalangeal joint of the big toe, which sometimes becomes painful just after operative correction of this malposition of the first metatarsophalangeal joint. A painful hyperextension of the interphalangeal joint may occur, when the rheumatoid inflammation of the first metatarsophalangeal joint results in a hallux rigidus.

I hope that it was possible to illucidate the most common examples not only of interplay between hindfoot and forefoot, but also between neighbouring joints in the course of rheumatoid disease of the foot.

References

Dwyer, F.C.: Osteotomy of the calcaneum for pes cavus. J. Bone Jt Surg. *41B:* 80–86 (1956).

Evans, D.: Calcaneo-valgus deformity. J. Bone Jt. Surg. *57B:* 270–278 (1975).

Hohmann, G.: Fuss und Bein: Ihre Erkrankungen und deren Behandlung; 4th ed. (Bergmann, München 1948).

Kirkup, J.R.: Ankle and tarsal joints in rheumatoid arthritis. Scand. J. Rheum. *3:* 50–52 (1974).

Tillmann, K.: The rheumatoid foot. Diagnosis, pathemechanics and treatment (Thieme, Stuttgart 1979).

Vahvanen, V.: Arthrodesis of the TC or pantalar joints in rheumatoid arthritis. Acta orthop. scand. *40:* 642–652 (1969).

Vainio, K.: The rheumatoid foot: a clinical study with pathological and roentgenological comments. Annls Chir. Gynaec. Fenn. *45:* suppl. 1 (1956).

Prof. Dr. med. K. Tillmann, Orthopädische Abteilung der Rheumaklinik
Bad Bramstedt GmbH, D-2357 Bad Bramstedt (FRG)

Rheumatology, vol. 11, pp. 100–103 (Karger, Basel 1987)

Operative Treatment with Special Regard to the Hindfoot

Anders Wigren

Department of Orthopaedic Surgery, University Hospital, Uppsala, Sweden

Hindfoot involvement is common in rheumatoid arthritis. In Vainio's [1956] material the talocrural joint was involved in 9% and the subtalar joints in 70%. Gschwend [1977] found an overall involvement of the ankle joint in 52% out of 300 cases. Unfortunately pain in the ankle and tenosynovitis at both malleolei are often not recognized as caused by synovitis and joint destruction of the subtalar joints, or more specified the talonavicular, the talocalcanear and the calcaneocuboidal joints. Roentgenographic signs of arthritis in the talocrural joint are most often registered but the more discrete roentgenological changes in the subtalar joints are more seldom notified. Varus or valgus malposition of the foot is more often caused by secondary deformation of the loose type of the subtalar joints or a result of osteoporosis than caused by changes in the talocrural joint. The varus or valgus malposition will appear at the same time as the rheumatoid flat foot develops. Such a deformity strongly influences the whole leg. Even severe deformities of the talocrural joint can be accepted if the foot is plantigrad [Gschwend, 1977]. For the same reason it is recommended to correct and stabilize the subtalar joints before a talocrural arthroplasty is performed [Pahle, personal communication].

Arthrodesis of the talocalcanear, talonavicular and calcaneocuboidal joints is often called triple arthrodesis but subtalar arthrodesis might be a better word. Usually in Scandinavia we have looked upon these three joints as a communicating system and arthrodeses of all three joints have usually been performed in rheumatoid arthritis when surgery has been indicated.

Patients and Methods

Twenty-five subtalar arthrodeses in 21 patients with rheumatoid arthritis were performed at the Orthopaedic Department, Uppsala, between 1973 and 1984. The age at the operation varied between 16 and 73 years with a mean of 50 years.

The indications for surgery were pain with or without synovitis at the ankle. The pain was often severe when walking on a rough ground. Further indications were varus or valgus deformity with pains and stabilization of the subtalar area before an arthroplasty of the talocrural joint was performed. Conservative measurements including a Lange support or an orthosis had not been found helpful or was not accepted by the patient. The feet operated on could be divided into two groups preoperatively. One with a normal mechanical axis and just disappearance of the joint space or just breaking of the longitudinal arch. This group included nine feet. The other appeared with dislocation in varus or valgus and included the loose unstable rheumatoid foot described by Clayton. This group included 16 feet. Twelve of these were suggested an ankle joint arthroplasty as a secondary operation. A triple arthrodesis was performed in all cases and a triplane osteotomy was done in all feet with a varus or valgus deformity. The arthrodesis was stabilized with staples and a plaster of Paris cast was applied for 10–12 weeks. A well supporting shoe was then used for a long time. Full weight bearing was allowed as soon as the patient was able to do so. The follow-up varied between half a year and 11 years with a mean of 4.5 years.

Results

Roentgenographically most arthrodeses were consolidated at 4 months. Bony consolidation of the talonavicular joint was delayed in 6 out of 25 feet but there was bony consolidation in all feet without further intervention. All feet with varus or valgus deformity were fully corrected to a good mechanical axis. Only four feet out of the twelve with a planned ankle joint replacement had such a discomfort left after the subtalar arthrodesis that they got their replacement. Concerning pain, all got rid of their pain. It is obvious that an evaluation of the four who had an ankle joint replacement after the subtalar arthrodesis was impossible. There were no major complications. Four local infections with delayed wound healing were well controlled with antibiotics and as soon as the arthrodesis was consolidated no further problem appeared.

Discussion

Subtalar arthrodesis in rheumatoid arthritis seems to be a very good pain-relieving procedure in the hands of the surgeons who favour this method. Once we recognize the symptoms, the painful arthritis of the subtalar joints is easy to find and separate from arthritis of the talocrural joint. Most of the pain in the hindfoot in rheumatoid arthritis seems to come from the subtalar joints and not from the talocrural joint. Thus triple arthrodesis can reduce the need for an arthroplasty of the talocrural joint. In our own material only one third of the patients suggested an ankle joint replacement needed this procedure once their subtalar joint had been corrected and fused. An ankle joint replacement on an unstable or tilted hindfoot can be expected to be an early problem and subtalar arthrodesis must be looked upon as the first step in planning for an ankle joint replacement. The postoperative treatment in a plaster cast could be a real problem for the rheumatoid patient with severe arm deformities. In planning for the procedure it seems necessary to consider this and to have a plan for the social service of the patient during the healing period.

Conclusion

The subtalar joints are very often involved in the biomechanics of the whole leg. Especially today when we are performing a lot of knee arthroplasties the knee and foot deformity must be looked upon together as a combined entity. The subtalar joints have a strong influence on the mechanical axis of the leg and are often the course of severe pain at the ankle. In planning for ankle joint arthroplasty it is necessary to have a well balanced and pain-free subtalar joint. The rheumatoid inflammation sooner or later will involve all three subtalar joints and therefore it is recommended to perform a triple arthrodesis and not an isolated arthrodesis of just the talonavicular joint. Triple or subtalar arthrodesis seems to be a safe procedure which is pain relieving, can improve the mechanical axis of the leg and in our material also seems to reduce the need for ankle joint procedures.

References

Gschwend, N.: Die operative Behandlung der chronischen Polyarthritis; 2nd ed. (Thieme, Stuttgart 1977).

Tillmann, K.: The rheumatoid foot (Thieme, Stuttgart 1979).

Vainio, K.: The rheumatoid foot: a clinical study with pathological and roentgenological comments. Annls Chir. Gynaec. Fenn. *45:* suppl. 1 (1956).

Anders Wigren, MD, Department of Orthopaedic Surgery, University Hospital, S-751 85 Uppsala (Sweden)

Rheumatology, vol. 11, pp. 104–113 (Karger, Basel 1987)

Ankle Arthrodesis

A Material of 148 Ankle Fusions on 130 Ankle Joints of 118 Patients

Vappu Uuspää, Pauli Raunio

Rheumatism Foundation Hospital, Hamina, Finland

Materials and Methods

The material consists of 148 ankle fusions on 130 ankle joints performed by several surgeons in the Rheumatism Foundation Hospital during the years 1955–81. 25% of the operations were performed by Prof. K. Vainio, another 25% by Dr. H. Laine, and the remaining 50% by 11 other surgeons. The material included 9 pantalar fusions. In 2 cases talocalcanear, in one case Chopart joint, and in one case talonavicular joint fusion was combined to the talocrural fusion.

The 130 ankle joints were re-examined 8 months to 27 years after the arthrodesis operation. The average follow-up was 8 years. There were 118 patients, 94 female, age 17–66, mean 45 years, and 24 male, age 32–63, mean 50 years. 90% of the patients were unemployable, 2 of them in wheel-chair.

Duration of the rheumatoid disease which was rheumatoid arthritis in 105 cases and juvenile chronic arthritis in 11 cases was 2–46 years, mean 16 years. The disease was polyarthritic in 114 and oligoarthritic in 2 cases, and clinically active in 73% of the cases. Erythrocyte sedimentation rate (ESR) ranged from 3 to 121, average 43.

Medical treatment at the time of the arthrodesis was gold in 53 cases, antimalarial treatment in 30, glucocorticoids in 34, salicylates in 69, indomethacin in 53 (in 17 out of the 33 non-union cases), phenylbutazone in 47, and 6 other 'rheuma medicines' in 12 cases.

The rheumatoid ankle joints, 71 right and 57 left, had been involved 1–46 years, on average 13 years before the arthrodesis. In addition there was one case of ankle tuberculosis and one instable fractura trigoni posterior tibiae.

Considering previous surgery of the other joints of the limb 24% had had total hip replacement, 20% total knee replacement, 8% knee fusion, 20% other knee operation, *70% subtalar/triple fusion*, and 47% forefoot operations.

Operative Techniques

Several operative techniques were used, resulting in 33 non-unions per 148 operations, 22%.

Compression arthrodesis modo Laine, 29 cases, gave the lowest, 14% pseudarthrosis rate: *Anterolateral incisions;* an inch of the tip of the lateral malleolus was resected, the talocrural joint and the distal tibiofibular syndemosis were chiselled; no internal fixation; compression apparatus 4–7 weeks, and then walking plaster cast 3–12 weeks (fig. 1). Anterior arthrodesis gave 4 non-unions per 18 operations, 22%. Anterior arthrodesis with iliac crest bone graft resulted in 2 non-unions (both reoperations) per 11 fusions, 9 out of which were reoperations (fig. 2).

Transfibular arthrodesis modo Vainio, 25 cases, lateral *oblique* incision, had 20% pseudarthrosis rate; with one screw and compression apparatus added 17% (fig. 4). Transfibular arthrodesis with lateral longitudinal incision, 65 cases, had 31% pseudarthrosis rate: 43 cases with one screw/screws on either tibial or talar side, 30% (fig. 5); 34 cases with one screw and compression apparatus, 32%; 20 cases with screws on both tibial and talar side, 45% pseudarthrosis rate. Considering operative wound scars, 75% looked like healed per primam intentionem. The percentage of unsatisfactory scars was the same 25 also in properly consolidated fusions.

Results

Patients Opinion

There was improvement in 113 cases and no improvement in 6 cases. 83 patients had some inconvenience of the stiff ankle joint, 39 patients had not, 93 patients would have had the operation again, 14 would not. The rest of the patients did not answer the questions.

Solid Ankle Fusion, 109 Ankle Joints

Pain: 80% had no pain
6% had night pain
12% had pain on movement
14% had pain on weight-bearing
Footwear: 50% wore normal shoes
8% needed insoles
15% needed shoelift
13% needed special shoes
Motion: 53% were able to walk 1 km at least
24% walked about 500 m (fig. 6)
19% walked 100 m at most
3% indoors only
2% were unable to walk
70% limped
60% needed no support
10% were unable to walk stairs
7% were able to run (fig. 3)

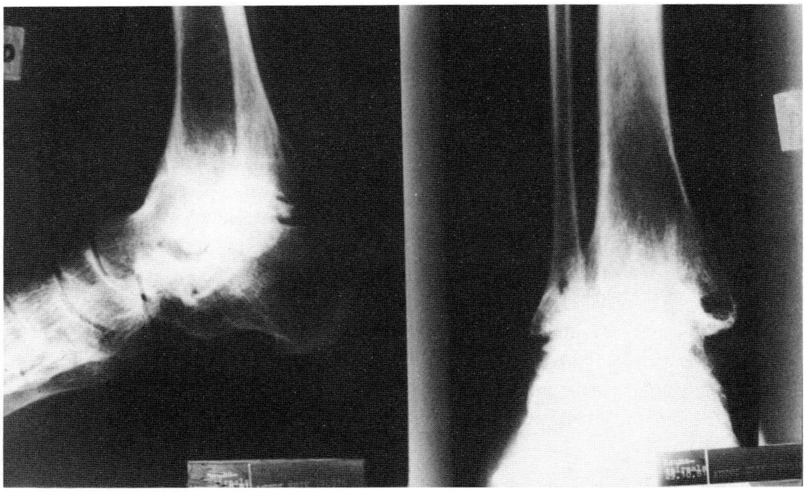

a

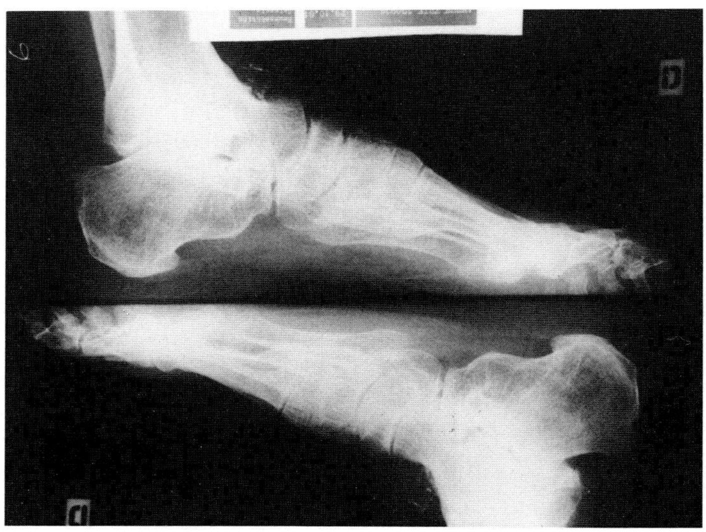

b

Fig. 1. a, b A male patient, age 60. Seropositive RA 17 years. Active polyarthritis. Ankle joint involved 1 year and treated previously by several intra-articular glucocorticoid injections. Antimalarial-glucocorticoid-salicylate medication. In addition 22 years previously cochleofixatio fracturae bimalleolaris. Re-examination 4 years 7 months after compression arthrodesis modo Laine: The patient wore normal shoes and was able to walk more than 1 km. No inconvenience. Solid ankle fusion in 15° valgus position with compensatory flexion movement from Chopart joint.

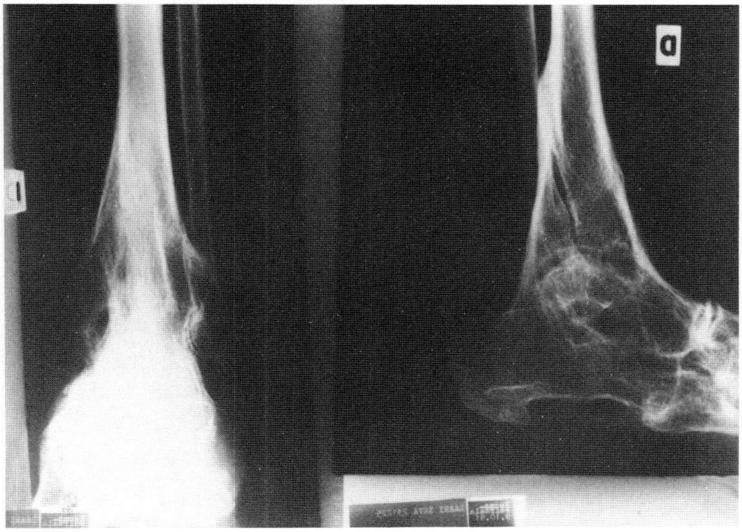

Fig. 2. A female patient, age 29. JCA 17 years, active polyarthritis. Ankle joint involved 17 years. No medical treatment. Re-examination 25 years 10 months after anterior arthrodesis with iliac crest graft. No pain. The patient wears insoles and is able to walk 2 km. Solid fusion in 10° equinus position.

Physical Examination

Position. 77% were in the valgus position up to 25°, average 5°. 12% were in neutral, and 11% in varus up to 15°, average 5°. 60% of the joints were in the equinus position up to 30°, average 10°. 29% were in the neutral position. 11% were in the dorsiflexion position up to 15° (1 case with meningomyelocele and spastic paresis in addition), average 5°. 50% were in the external rotation position up to 20°, average 10°. 32% were in the neutral position. 18% were internally rotated up to 15°, average 5°. 60% of the fused ankle joints looked deformed. 67% had pes planus deformity in addition. 49% had callosities. 57% had swollen legs, 73% of the painful cases. 69% had calf atrophy, 81% of the pain cases. 6% had pain on flexion stress, 7% on supination stress. 57% had a shortening of the leg from 1 to 11 cm, average 2 cm; 37%

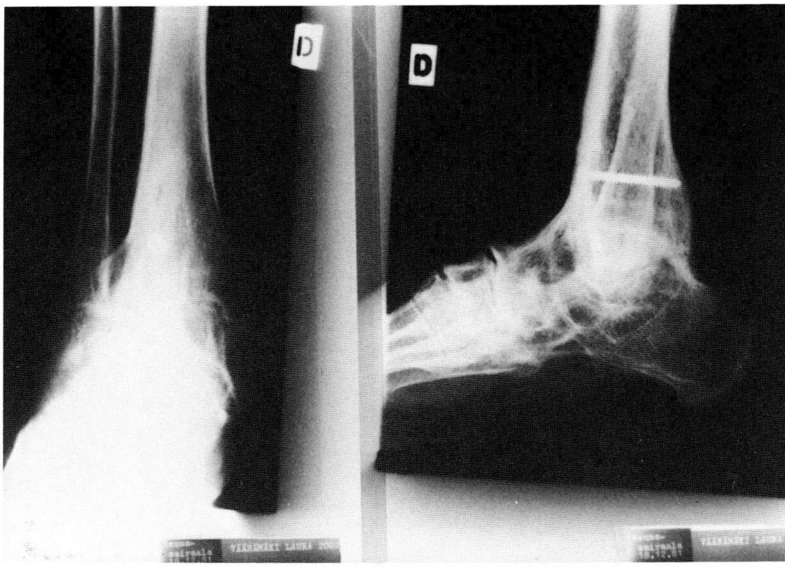

Fig. 3. A female patient, age 36. Seropositive RA 15 years, active polyarthritis. Ankle joint involved 12 years and previously treated with intra-articular glucocorticoid injections. Gold and antimalarial treatment at the time of the operation. Re-examination 17 years 7 months after anterior arthrodesis with tibial graft fixed with one screw. No pain, no inconvenienc. The patient works as a janitor, wears normal shoes. Learned to run 7 years after operation and had continued jogging 10 years. Solid fusion in 5° valgus, 5° equinus and 10° external rotation position.

1 cm, 12% 2 cm, 6% 3 cm, and 2% up to 11 cm. 60% had compensatory tarsal flexion movement up to 40°, average 10°. Tarsal pro-supination movement was absent in 20%, and restricted to 20° on average with solid ankle fusion, and to 15° with solid pantalar fusion.

Radiological Findings

X-Ray showed in 17% a mere solid ankle fusion, in 57% solid pantalar fusion, and in 13% solid bony fusion to the toes was seen.

Analysis of the Pseudarthrosis Cases

Besides the operative methods the non-union cases were compared with the properly consolidated considering the disease itself, the medical treatment, previous operative treatment, etc. Few differences were

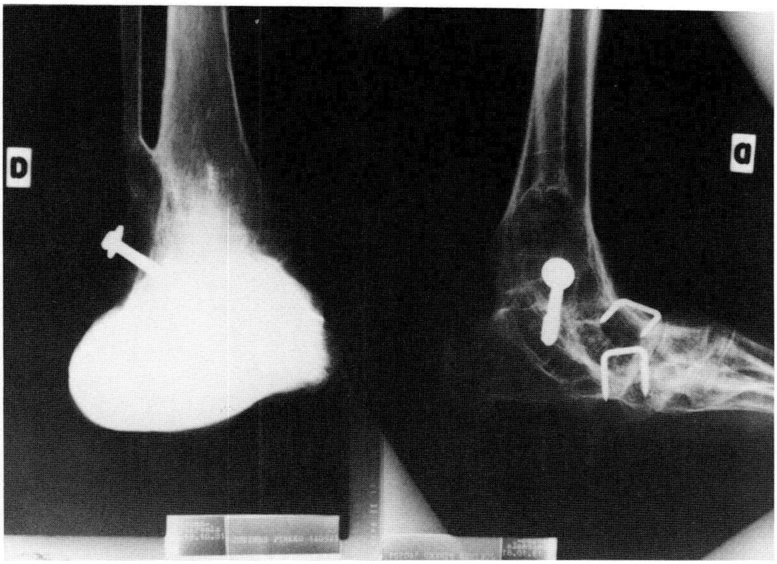

Fig. 4. A female patient, age 48. Seronegative RA 12 years, active polyarthritis. Ankle joint involved 7 years. Salicylate medication. Subtalar arthrodesis 3 years previously. Re-examined 11 years 6 months after transfibular arthrodesis modo Vainio. No pain. Wore normal shoes and was able to walk 2 km at least. Solid fusion in 10° valgus, 5° dorsiflexion and 5° internal rotation.

noted. In each group one out of five patients was male with the same average age. One out of 10 had juvenile disease. The average durations of the disease was 16.5 years in non-unions compared with 15.5 years in consolidated cases. There was one oligoarticular case in each group. 9 out of 10 non-unions and 7 out of 10 consolidated ones had seropositive disease. 8 out of 10 of the former and 7 out of 10 of the latter had a clinically active disease, but the average ESR was 35 and 45, respectively. Considering medical treatment gold was given equally often, antimalarial treatment but half as frequently in the non-union cases. One out of 5 non-unions and 1 out of 3 consolidated ones had glucocorticoids, one out of 10 in each group every other day. There was one case with cytostatic treatment in each group. One half of the patients had salicylates in each group. One out of two non-unions and one out of three consolidated ones had indomethacin. One third had phenylbutazone in each group. Before the ankle arthrodesis the non-union

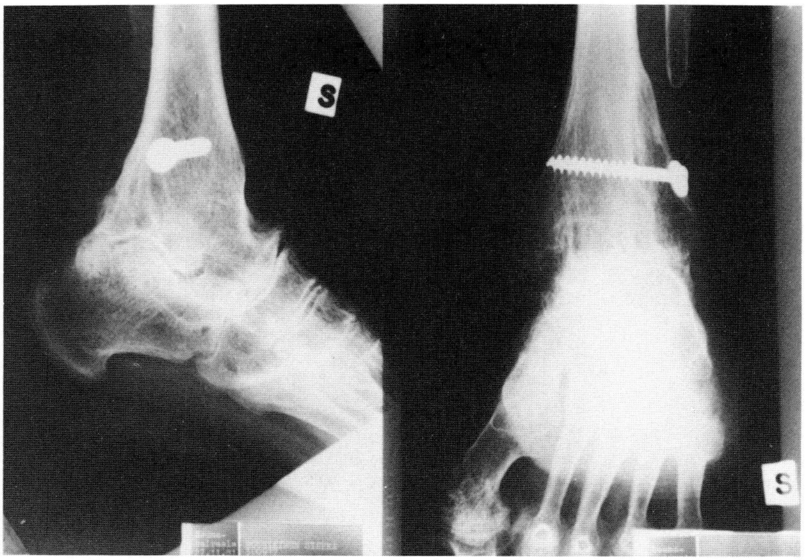

Fig. 5. A female patient, age 58. Seronegative RA 32 years. Inactive polyarthritis. Ankle joint involved 32 years. No medication. Re-examination 5 years 10 months after transfibular arthrodesis with lateral longitudinal incision along fibula and one screw to tibia. Solid union in 20° equinus position to be able to wear high heel shoes. She regretted that the operation had not been done 10 years earlier already.

patients had been operated on 0–30 times each, average 10 times, the consolidated ones 0–32 times each, average 8 times. 4% of the previous operations had been infected in the non-union group and 5% of the operations of the consolidated ones.

There were *fewer previous operations of the other joints of the limb with non-union* ankle joint: THR 13% compared with 27% in the consolidated ones; no TKR nor knee arthrodesis, compared with 23 and 8%, respectively, in the consolidated ones (31% other knee operations, 19% in the latter group).

Subtalar/triple fusion was more frequent, 79/69%, respectively. Forefoot operations were equal 46 and 48%, respectively. One ankle joint with previous Erbium* synovectomy had ankle fusion twice, resulting in non-union. In both groups 6% had had surgical synovectomy. 18% of the non-unions and 13% of the consolidated were reoperations.

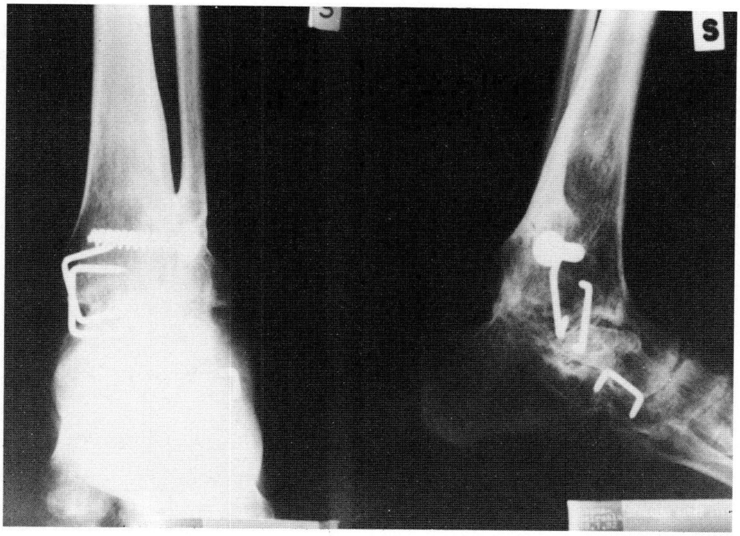

Fig. 6. A female patient, age 22. Seronegative RA 3 years. Active polyarthritis. Ankle joint involved 1 year. Antimalarial-glucocorticoid-phenylbutazone treatment. Reexamination 10 years 6 months after transfibular arthrodesis modo Vainio, 9 years 5 months after corrective osteotomy to diminish 15° valgus position, and 6 months after ICLH arthroplasty of the other ankle joint. She is mathematics teacher working normally at school. 'There is starting pain in the prosthesis ankle, in the fused one none', was her comment.

Discussion

In the present material the simplest method, modo Laine, with no internal fixation material seems to have given the lowest pseudarthrosis rate. The more internal fixation material the higher pseudarthrosis rate.

In Vahvanen's [1969] material of 32 arthrodesis of TC and pantalar joints from Rheumatism Foundation Hospital the pseudarthrosis rate was 19%. The operations performed by the methods of Guildal and Sodemann [1930], Adams [1948], and Charnley [1951] were successful. Pseudarthrosis occurred after anterior arthrodesis with iliac crest graft. The cases of latter method included in the present material seem to have a more favourable result compared to the transfibular approach with longitudinal incision.

When compared with other previously published materials the results of the present rheumatoid ankle material closely resemble those of Lance et al. [1971], though their material mainly consisted of poliomyelitis and trauma cases; only 8 out of 183 patients had rheumatoid arthritis. Our overall non-union rate is the same 22%. The non-union rate is lowest with compression arthrodesis, by us modo Laine, in their material modo Charnley. In their material factors relating to poor results were technical errors, neurological disorders, heterogeneous bone grafts, a transfibular operative approach and associated triple arthrodesis. In the present material 70% of the cases had a previous subtalar/triple arthrodesis, but its role in relation to non-unions is less clear.

60% of the cases had compensatory tarsal flexion movement. The percentage was but slightly higher, 64, in cases that caused no inconvenience to the patient. Instead those limbs had fewer previous operations of hip, knee, and forefoot region.

Summary

The material consists of 148 ankle fusions on 130 ankle joints of 118 patients, performed by 13 surgeons during the years 1955–81, and re-examined 8 months to 27 years after operation, the average follow-up 8 years.

There were 33 pseudarthrosis per 148 operations, 22%. Compression arthrodesis modo Laine, anterolateral incision, no internal fixation, gave the lowest, 14% pseudarthrosis rate. Anterior arthrodesis had 22% pseudarthrosis rate; with iliac crest graft 18%. Transfibular arthrodesis modo Vainio, lateral oblique incision, had 20% pseudarthrosis rate; with one screw and compression apparatus 17%. Transfibular arthrodesis with lateral longitudinal incision had 31% pseudarthrosis rate: with one screw/screws on either tibial or talar side 30%; with one screw and compression apparatus 32%; with screws on both tibial and talar side 45% pseudarthrosis rate.

With solid ankle fusions, 109 joints, 77% were in the valgus position, average 5°; 60% in equinus, average 10°; 50% in external rotation position, average 10°. 60% had compensatory tarsal flexion movement up to 40°, average 10°.

References

Adams, J.C.: Arthrodesis of the ankle. Experiences with the transfibular approach. J. Bone Jt Surg. *30B:* 506 (1948).

Charnley, J.: Compression arthrodesis of the ankle and shoulder. J. Bone Jt Surg. *33B:* 180 (1951).

Guildal, P.; Sodemann, T.: Result of 256 triarticular arthrodesis of the foot in sequelae of infantile paralysis. Acta orthop. scand. *1:* 199 (1930).
Lance, E.M.; Pavel, A.; Patterson, R.L., Jr.; Fries, L.; Larsen, I.J.: Arthrodesis of the ankle; a follow-up study. J. Bone Jt Surg. *53A:* 1030 (1971).
Vahvanen, V.: Arthrodesis of the tc or pantalar joints in rheumatoid arthritis. Acta orthop. scand. *40:* 642 (1969).

Vappu Uuspää, MD, Rheumatism Foundation Hospital, Murtalhontie 279, SF-49420 Hamina 2 (Finland)

Rheumatology, vol. 11, pp. 114–125 (Karger, Basel 1987)

Stable Fixation in Hindfoot Arthrodesis, a Valuable Procedure in the Complex RA Foot

N. Gschwend, U. Steiger

Klinik Wilhelm Schulthess, Zürich, Schweiz

In a survey of 300 rheumatoid arthritic patients with an average duration of the disease of 10 years, we found the ankle and subtalar joints being involved in 52%. This is very much less frequent than the involvement of the forefeet. Vainio [1a, b] already stated that radiological changes are to be seen relatively late, on average 7 years after the beginning of the disease. Tillmann [2] found that only 5–10% of all the patients showed the initial symptoms at the level of the rear foot. In contrast to this, the juvenile rheumatoid arthritis frequently starts at the level of the ankle joints (according to Böni [3] in 68%). From a functional point of view the involvement of the ankle joint is certainly of less importance than that of the knee or the hip joint. Walking capacity is rarely jeopardized by ankle joint involvement. Moreover, there is a possibility for functional compensation by the neighboring joints or by shoe adaptations. The most frequent deformity of the rear foot is a valgus deformity, which according to Vahvanen [4] is to be found in more than 80% of adult rheumatoid arthritis with rear foot involvement. Varus deformity is relatively seldom, around 10% in adults, but more frequent in juveniles (33%). The cavus foot is rare (less than 10%).

Taking our own statistics we found in a survey compiled in 1981 that out of a total of 4,700 operations performed in rheumatoid arthritis, the ankle joint was operated only in 79, whereas the forefoot in 323. This confirms what has just been said. Mostly there is a discrepancy between the clinical and radiological picture, in the sense that the symptoms even in more advanced radiological changes can be considered of

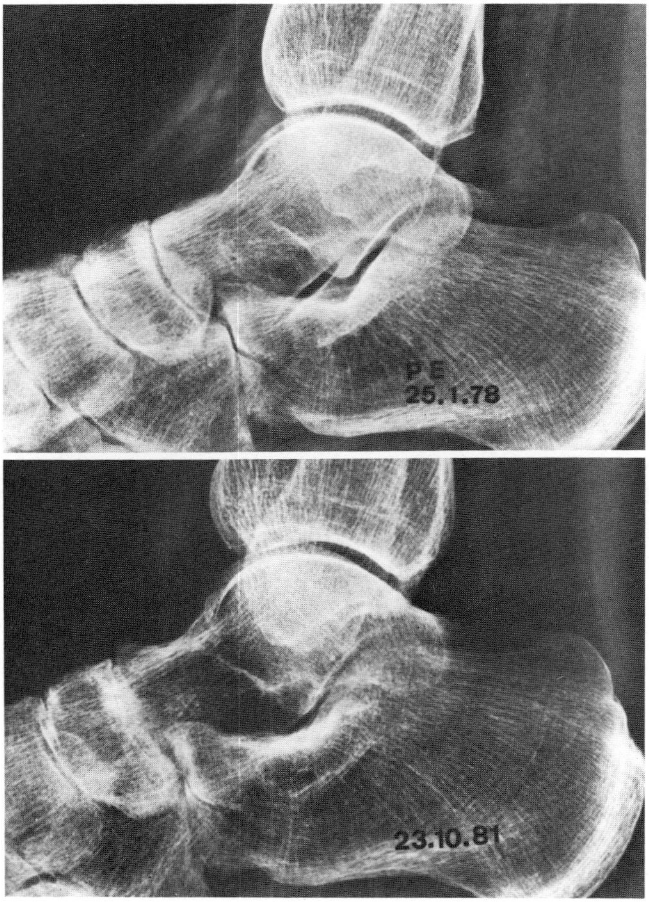

Fig. 1. Taloscaphoid joint involvement may mimic ankle joint involvement.

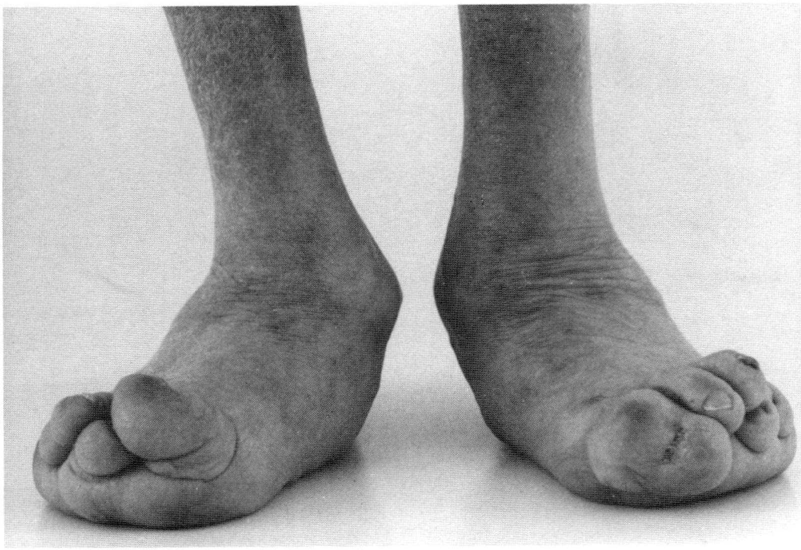

Fig. 2. Typical RA foot deformity: Valgus of the hind foot, forefoot with dislocated metatarsophalangeal joints, plantar bursitis and hammer toes.

minor importance. The relatively frequent involvement of the taloscaphoid joint may mimic an ankle joint involvement (fig. 1).

Figure 2 shows the most frequent deformity in the rheumatoid arthritic foot: valgus deformity of the hind foot combined with a typical forefoot deformity. Figure 3 and 4 show that the valgus deformity may have its cause at the level of the subtalar joint or at the ankle joint. For definition of the various grades of involvement we are using the Larsen-Dale-Eek [5] (LDE) classification (fig. 5).

Therapeutical Considerations

In the LDE stages 0–3 we are favoring synovectomy provided that pain and swelling cannot be relieved by conservative methods. In stages 4 and 5 arthroplasty or arthrodesis have to be discussed, when symptoms resist the conservative treatment. Generally speaking, it can be said that in those countries where the art of the orthopedic shoemaker is highly developed, we will find less frequently surgical operations of the hindfoot.

In our view, *arthroplasty* of the *ankle joint* is still in an experimental phase and has too many complications. Moreover, it is not easily retrievable. On the other hand, the alternative, namely arthrodesis, gives such satisfactory results that we prefer doing an arthrodesis right away. The prerequisite is a good technique which allows a safe solid fusion in a short time and without being forced to fix the foot of the handicapped rheumatoid patients in a plaster cast for a longer period. The technique of Charnley [6] with the compression clamps gave us satisfaction in many cases, but in severe osteoporosis we saw the migration of the clamps and as a consequence late union or even non-union. Moreover, the risk of nailtrack infection is always present until the nails are removed. During this period the patient can be sent home only with difficulties and on the condition that a careful observation of the nailtrack is guaranteed.

Results of Compression Arthrodeses (Charnley Method)

Some years ago, we analyzed the results of 21 consecutive cases in which we performed a Charnley [6] compression arthrodesis of the ankle joint. There were 17 female and 4 male patients. All were seropositive and had a polyarthritic involvement of most joints. In these 21 patients, we arthrodesed 28 ankle joints, 17 on the right foot and 11 on the left foot. The influence on pain and swelling is shown in table I. The final qualifications of the operation by the patient and by the surgeon can be seen in table II. In conclusion, we can see that the results of ankle fusion was very satisfactory already with the method presented.

Wagner's Method of Hindfoot Fusion

The wish to get a bony fusion in a shorter time and to be able to dispense with nails perforating the skin with the risk of infection or migration in the bone and finally to facilitate after-treatment, led us to

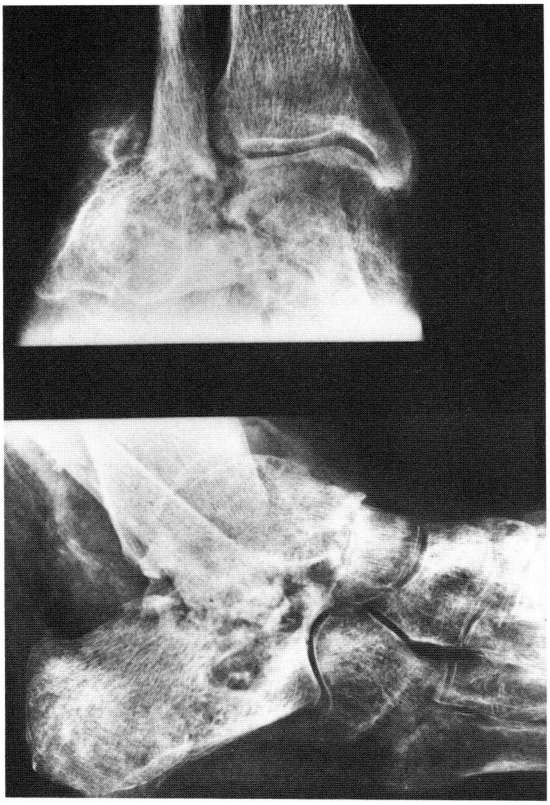

Fig. 3. Valgus foot due to destruction of the subtalar joint.

adopt *Wagner's method* of ankle subtalar or pantalar fusion. The incision is shown in figure 6. The technique is extensively described in the publication of Wagner and Puck [7]. For subtalar fusion we are normally using two compression screws (fig. 7). For the ankle fusion we normally are also using two screws (fig. 8). The two little screws seen in figure 8 have nothing to do with the fixation of the ankle joint, but fix only the fibula to the tibia and talus serving as a graft. This is a modification of Wagner's method, who normally does not osteotomize the malleoli. We found this technique easier than the original technique.

Fig. 4. Valgus foot due to destruction of the ankle joint.

Fig. 5. Larsen-Dale-Eek (LDE) grades of ankle destruction in RA.

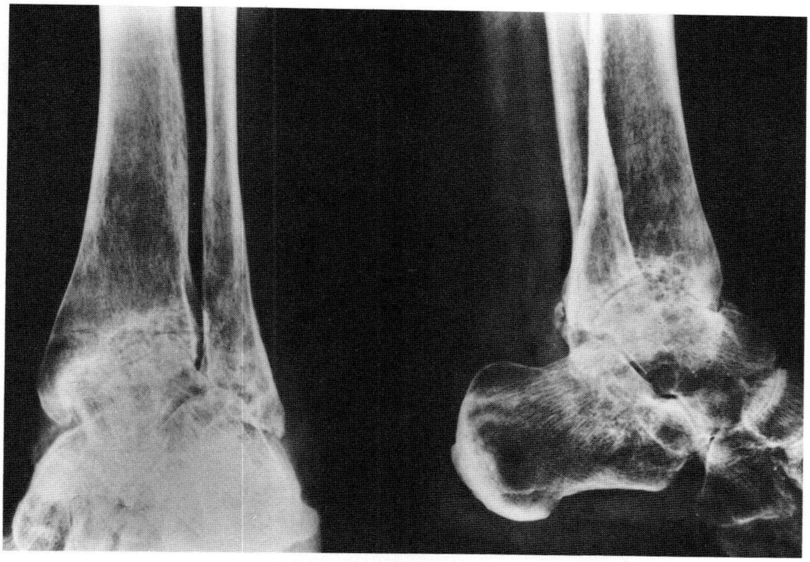

4

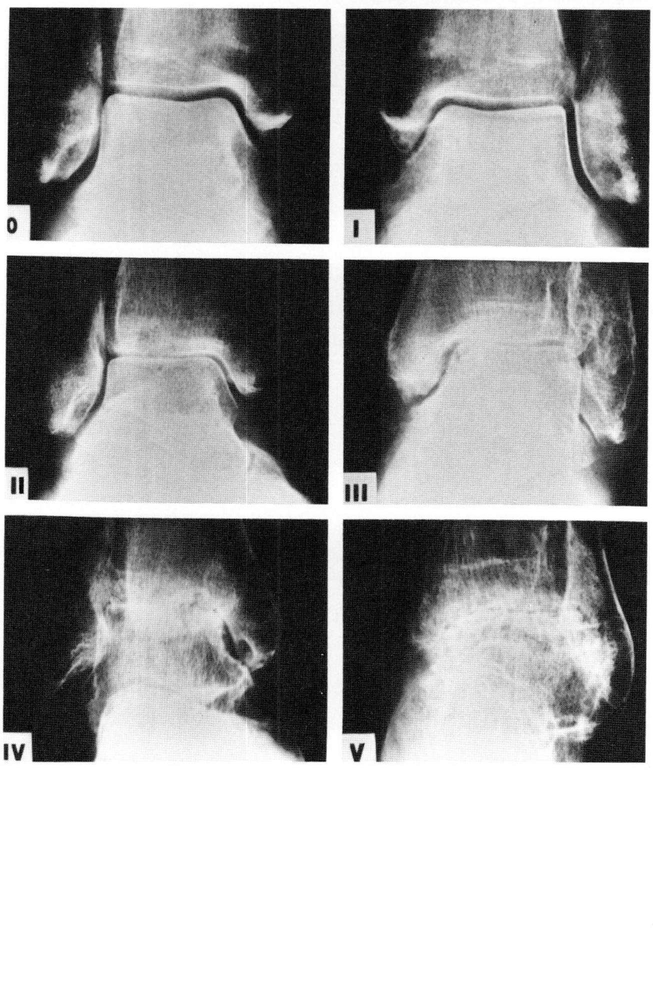

5

Table I. Results of arthrodesis

		Preop.	Postop.
Pain	none	0	21
	slight	0	0
	severe	28	1
Swelling	none	4	18
	slight	13	8
	severe	11	2

Table II. Results of arthrodesis

Final qualification	By the patient	By the surgeon
Good	23	23
Satisfactory	5	4
Poor	0	1

For the fusion of the ankle and subtalar joints (fig. 9) or for pantalar arthrodesis (fig. 10) three screws suffice, provided we fix the Chopart joint with staples or compression screws. For the screw which goes from the tibia to the talus, it is important to make a special slot in the tibia, where the washer can be placed in such a way that it serves as a resistant base for compression (fig. 11).

Results

We were able to analyze the results in 34 patients with 35 feet, 12 being male and 22 female patients. 12 concerned the left foot and 23 the right foot. The age ranged between 16 and 76, the average was 44.5 years (tables III and IV).

In this series the main indications were: osteoarthritis (table V), paralytic foot, rheumatoid arthritis, congenital club foot, sepsis and coalitio calcaneonavicularis.

6, 7

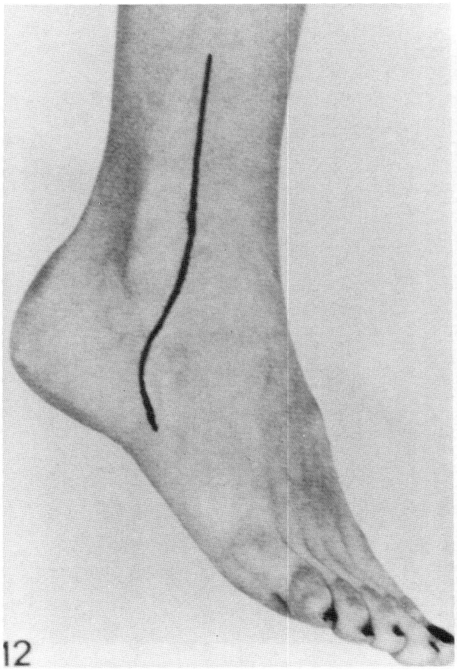

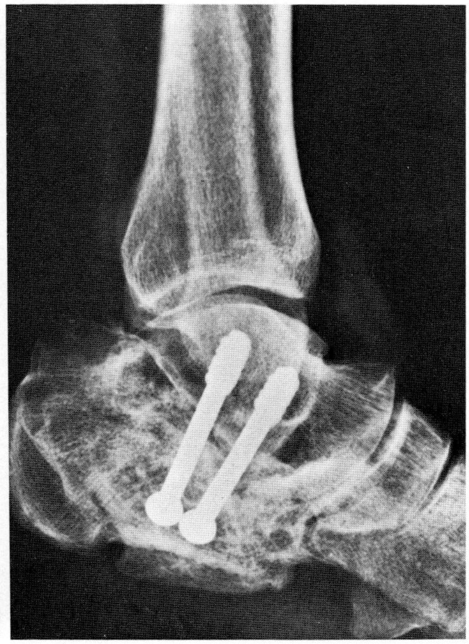

Fig. 6. Skin incision for Wagner's hind foot arthrodesis.
Fig. 7. Subtalar fusion with two compression screws.

Bony fusion was obtained in a much shorter time than with the previous methods. In 60% we found fusion after 8 weeks, and 97% after 12 weeks, on average after 9 weeks. The stay in hospital, which in the earlier cases lasted 5–6 weeks (until the nails and clamps could be removed and a plaster cast applied), has been significantly reduced; the average stay in hospital was 20 days (range 10–38 days). There is no doubt that the patients with this method of arthrodesis can be sent home after a couple of days, provided wound healing is supervized at regular intervals and the patient has sufficient personal care at home. The complication rate is low. Problems of wound healing are most frequent and are found in our statistic in 3 cases without lasting consequences. In 2 cases a lesion of a lateral skin nerve was observed without lasting discomfort.

In conclusion we can say that arthrodesis of the ankle joint or subtalar joint or pantalar arthrodesis is a most rewarding operation. Using

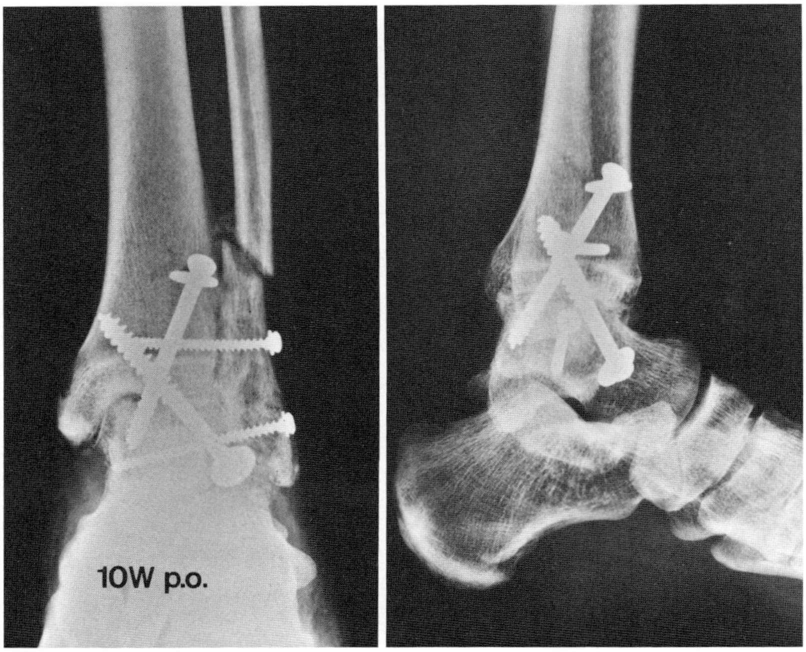

Fig. 8. Ankle fusion with two compression screws. The two little screws fix only the fibular graft.

Table III. Ankle fusion

34 patients	12	0	22	0
35 feet	12	left	23	right
Age	16–76 years			
Average	44.5 years			

Wagner's method with the compression screws, we get excellent compression between the fragments with a minimum risk of secondary deformity with an easy aftertreatment from a functional point of view and with a short stay in hospital. There is no doubt that this method is technically demanding. Eventually the metal has to be removed in a secondary procedure.

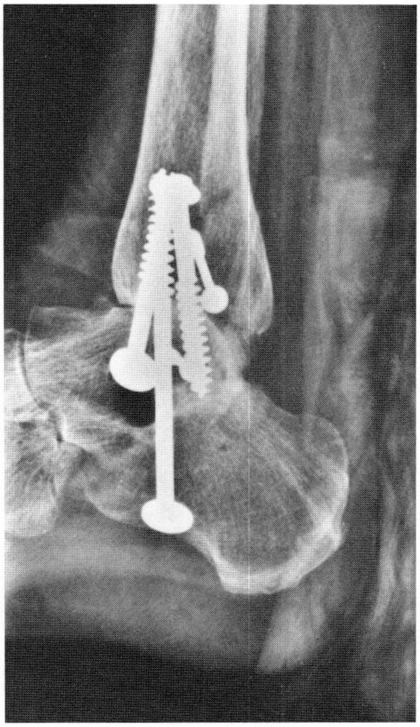

9

Fig. 9. Fusion of ankle and subtalar joint.
Fig. 10. Pantalar arthrodesis.

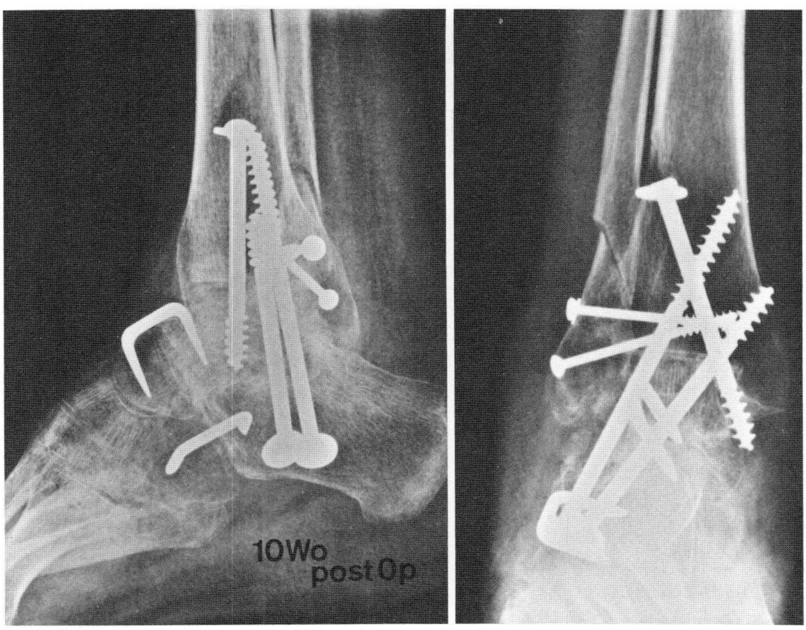

10

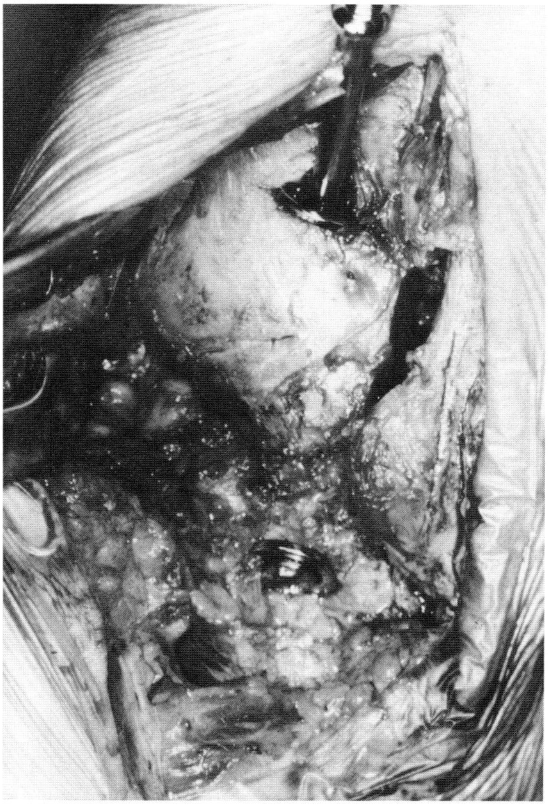

Fig. 11. Slot in the tibia to place the washer for the compression screw. Another screw fixes the talus to the tibia from distally to proximally.

Table IV. Ankle fusion (n = 35)

Operated joints	
Ankle fusion	13
Subtalar and chopart-joint fusion	11
Pantalar arthrodeses	5
Ankle and subtalar arthrodesis	4
Subtalar fusion	2

Table V. Indications (n = 35)

Osteoarthritis	15
Paralysis	8
Rheumatoid arthritis	5
Congenital clubfoot	3
Infection	2
Coalitio calcaneonaviculare	2

Table VI. Ankle fusion (n = 35)

	Time of consolidation, weeks
60%	8 weeks
97%	12 weeks
∅	9 weeks

Table VII. Ankle fusion (n = 35)

Hospitalization	10–38 days
∅	20 days

References

1a Vainio, K.: The rheumatoid foot. Annls Chir. Gynaec. Fenn. suppl. 1, p. 45 (1956).

1b Vainio, K.: The role of surgery on the rehabilitation of rheumatoid arthritis patients. Proc. 4th Eur. Rheum. Congr. (Istanbul Press, Istanbul 1959).

2 Tillmann, K.: Der rheumatische Fuss und seine Behandlung (Enke, Stuttgart 1977).

3 Böni, A.: Personal communication.

4 Vahvanen, V.: Arthrodesis of the TC or pantalar joints in rheumatoid arthritis. Acta orthop. scand. *40:* 642 (1969).

5 Larsen, A.; Dale, K.; Eek, M.: Radiographic evaluation of rheumatoid arthritis and related conditions by standard reference films. Acta radiol. (Diag.) *18:* 481 (1977).

6 Charnley, J.: Compression arthrodesis of the ankle and shoulder. J. Bone Jt Surg. *33B:* 180 (1951).

7 Wagner, H.; Puck, H.G.: Die Verschraubungsarthrodese der Sprunggelenke. Unfallheilkunde *85:* 280 (1982).

Prof. Dr. Norbert Gschwend, Klinik Wilhelm Schulthess,
Neumünsterallee 3, CH-8008 Zürich (Schweiz)

Rheumatology, vol. 11, pp. 126–130 (Karger, Basel 1987)

Synovectomy of MTP Joints in Rheumatoid Arthritis

A Preliminary Report

Heikki Aho

Department of Orthopedic Surgery, University Hospital, Tampere, Finland

Introduction

There are widely varying opinions about the role of synovectomy in rheumatoid arthritis (RA). However, it is one of the classic operations in the surgical treatment of RA [1]. It relieves pain and swelling and at least some authors believe in its prophylactic value [2, 3]. Metatarsophalangeal (MTP) joints are the most commonly affected ones in RA. Pain in the MTP joints often causes considerable difficulty in walking. Only one former preliminary report on the synovectomy of the MTP joints has been published. The author could report normalization of walking after synovectomy [4].

Patients and Methods

Since 1978 we have proposed MTP synovectomy for patients whose joints are not destroyed enough for the resection of the whole row, but still painful despite individually molded insoles and efficient medical treatment, intra-articular steroid included. The border between synovectomy and resection has been put between one and three badly eroded joints. If two joints are in bad condition, synovectomy is proposed only if the rest of the joints are better than Larsen grade 3 [5] (table I).

Table I. Present material

	Patients	Feet	Joints	Right/left
Female	11	16	57	28/29
Male	4	5	9	3/6

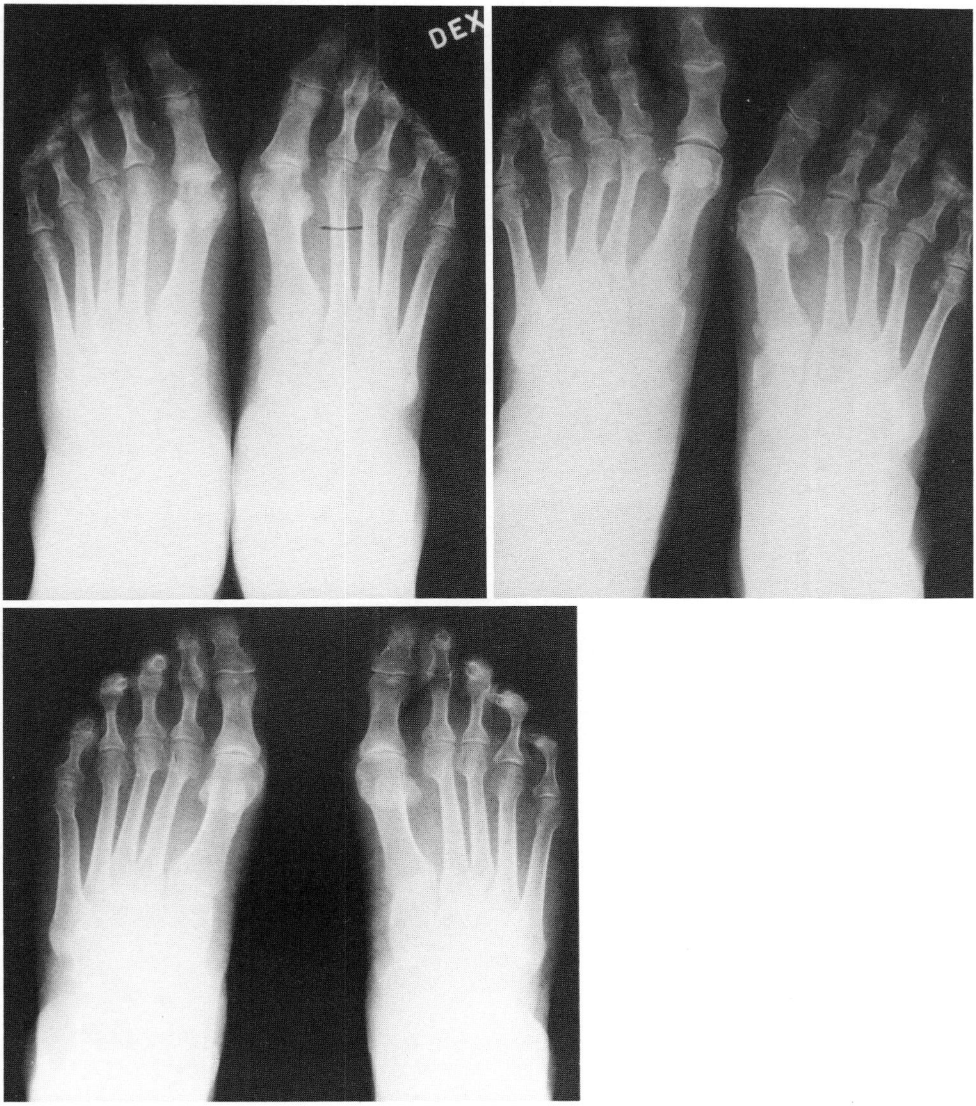

a *b* *c*

Fig. 1. Radiographic examples of synovectomized joints with excellent outcome: (a) joints I–V bilaterally; (b) joints I–V right and II–V left; (c) joints II–V right.

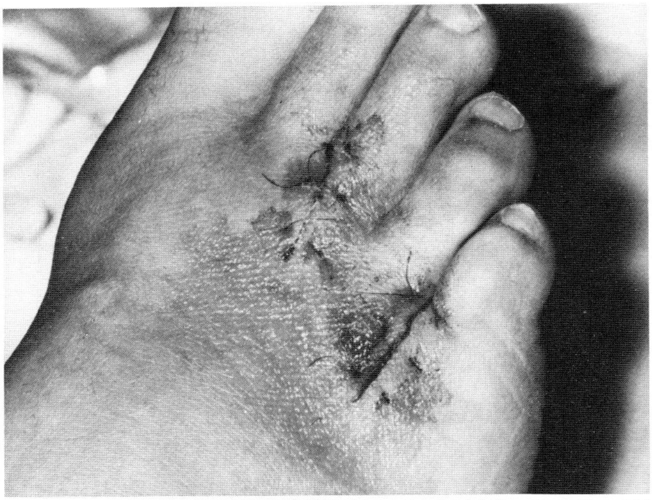

a

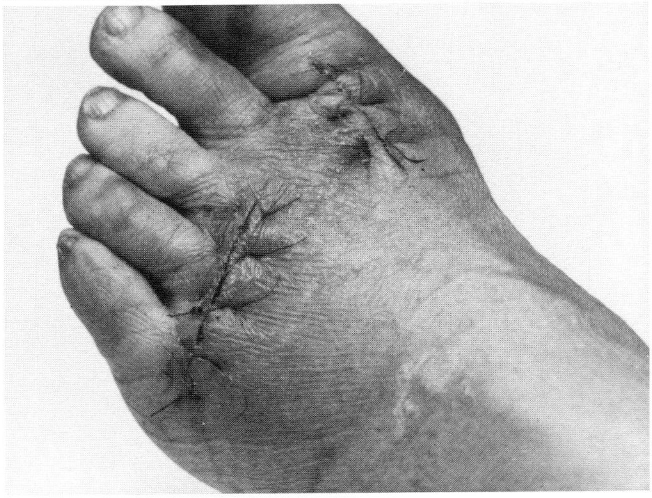

b

Fig. 2. Recommended incisions for the synovectomy of four (a) and five (b) MTP joints.

Every single symptomatic MTP joint has been synovectomized. Radiologically they range from normal to severely eroded. Only one or all five joints might be operated on. On average, three joints were synovectomized in one operation. Present material consists of the patients who have been followed-up at least one year. Dorsal longitudinal incisions have been used as a rule. Two neighbouring joints can be reached through one

Table II. Effect of the number of synovectomized joints on forefoot pain

Joints operated	Number of feet	Mean painless months (range)	Still symptom-free at follow-up
1-3	11	15 (0-48)	3
4-5	10	20 (6-72)	7
Total	21	18 (0-72)	10

incision. If not more than three neighbour joints are due to be operated on, a transverse dorsal incision has been used. Neither incision has produced any complications. The patients walk without aids the next day (fig. 1, 2).

Results

All but one patient became symptom-free. In the patient who did not benefit from synovectomy, a mistake was made. In addition to synovectomy of joints 2-4 the head of the fifth metatarsal was resected. She is also the only one with plantar incision (table II). The better result with four or five joints synovectomized is statistically not significant with so small figures.

Discussion

MTP synovectomy is easy to perform. Dorsal longitudinal as well as transverse incisions are harmless. Walking is corrected as far as it depends on painful MTP joints. Both feet can be operated on simultaneously.

Almost always a painless result can be achieved for months to years. In our patients only the totally pain-free period was registered. Partial pain relief is much longer. The data of my study does not allow conclusions, whether all (maybe first excluded, if not affected) or symptomatic joints only should be synovectomized.

References

1 Gschwend, N.: Indikationen zur Synovektomie bei chronischer Polyarthritis. Dt. med. Wschr. *110: 310–312* (1985).
2 Arthritis and Rheumatism Council and British Orthopaedic Association Report: Controlled trials of synovectomy of the knee and metacarpo-phalangeal joints in rheumatoid arthritis. Ann. rheum. Dis. *35:* 437–442 (1976).
3 Raunio, P.: Prophylactic value of synovectomy of the proximal interphalangeal finger joint in rheumatoid arthritis (academic dissertation). Scand. J. Rheumatol. suppl. 19 (1977).
4 Brattström, H.: Surgery in metatarsophalangeal joints II–V in rheumatoid arthritis. Acta orthop. belg. *38:* 107–113 (1972).
5 Larsen, A.; Dahle, K.; Eek, M.: Radiographic evaluation of rheumatoid arthritis and related conditions by standard reference films. Acta radiol. (Diag). *18:* 481–491 (1977).

Heikki Aho, MD, Tampere City Hospital, Hatanpää,
SF-33100 Tampere (Finland)

Rheumatology, vol. 11, pp. 131–135 (Karger, Basel 1987)

Midterm Results of Arthroplasty of the Forefoot by Clayton-Vainio in Rheumatoid Arthritis

H.J. Refior, R. Hoos

Orthopädische Klinik der Medizinischen Hochschule Hannover, Hannover, FRG

The area of the forefoot can be also one of the primary sites of rheumatoid arthritis [9] (16%). Gschwend [5] found that about 79% of his patients developed some kind of alteration of the forefoot after a 10-year course of that disease. He especially emphasizes the typical clinical picture of rheumatoid arthritis. Usually it consists of a displacement of the metatarsal heads downwards through the fat pad of the sole of the foot, so that they lie subcutaneously and tender callosities form under them. In addition the lateral 4 toes dislocate dorsally at the metatarsophalangeal joints and become clawed at the interphalangeal joints. The big toe usually develops a valgus deformity with bunions.

It was Vainio [13] who emphasized the fact that the pain caused stress-relieving position, in inflammatory diseases of the joints of the big toe, especially its metatarsophalangeal joint, is most important in the genesis of the rheumatoid pes planovalgus. In his opinion avoiding pressure to the painful big toe first leads to a deviation of the metatarsal bone and subsequently to a contract fixation in this position. As a result the forefoot and midfoot derotate [10, 12] and the long arch flattens. In the case where an additional fixation of the forefoot to a backfoot arises and the tibial edge of the foot returns to the ground, the backfoot necessarily returns into a pronation position, thus giving rise to a pes planovalgus.

Normally, the rheumatoid foot undergoes the same deforming mechanical stress as any other foot [7]. However, if pain and inflammation have led to muscle wasting, the mechanical stress is more impressive [11].

Tillmann [11] points at an amplifying effect: a rheumatoid hallux valgus can be the cause for alterations of the joints of the hindfoot which in itself is a mechanical cause for a deviation of the toes.

In addition to the mechanical component of the splayfoot, the destruction of the bursae and the metatarsophalangeal joints leads to a wearing of the plantar structures which leads to a dorsal luxation of the 4 lateral toes in their metatarsophalangeal joints. This causes a perforation of the metatarsal heads to the plantar side, thus giving the typical relief of rheumatoid forefoot with its profound skin callosities under each dislocated metatarsal head.

The complaints caused by these alterations of the forefoot including inflammatory components lead to the typical gait. During the whole phase of the step the patient tries to avoid any pressure on the forefoot. Because of this pathologically altered gait the other joints, that are afflicted by the same disease, become mechanically overstressed which gives rise to further destruction.

As early as 1912, Hoffmann [6] suggested a resection of the metatarsal head from the plantar side in these cases. This procedure has been applied and modified by various authors, last by Tillmann [8, 11]. In 1959, Fowler [4] used both a dorsal and a plantar incision.

In 1960, Clayton [3] described a dorsal approach resecting all the metatarsal heads and the bases of the toes. Especially important in this approach is the precise metatarsal index [1].

With reference to Barbier et al. [2], we also use a dorsal approach since August 1980, since these authors report a higher rate of complications when using a plantar approach. Furthermore, they report worse results using the plantar approach compared to the dorsal one. For the metatarsophalangeal joints of the great toe we prefer a separate approach according to Vainio [13] and for the toes II–V we use the technique given by Clayton [3].

For the after-treatment we recommend a postoperative compression treatment in a specially moulded plaster or plastic cast. The functional after-treatment of the toes starts 5 days postoperatively. After the healing of the wound and removal of the sutures on the 12th to the 14th day, the after-treatment consists of increasing pressure and gymnastics as well as support with stress-relieving insoles. The insoles should give good retrocapital support and a hallux night splint is used until the metatarsophalangeal joint of the big toe is stabilized.

Using these techniques, 117 feet have been operated upon at the Orthopedic Clinic of the MHH since August 1980. Considering a minimal convalescence time of 1 year, 98 feet could be reviewed for a period of 1–4 years, with an average of 2 years. In 35 cases the operation

Table I. Midterm results of arthroplasty of the forefoot by Clayton-Vainio in rheumatoid arthritis (n = 98)

Follow-up	1–4 years		average	2 years
Both sides	35		one side	28
Patients	63	women 57	men	6
Age	27–75		average	52

Table II. Midterm results of arthroplasty of the forefoot by Clayton-Vainio in rheumatoid arthritis (n = 98)

	Number	Percent
Primary healing	72	74
Necrosis of the skin	21	21
Infection	5	5

was performed on both sides. The 63 patients consisted of 57 women and 6 men. The age ranged from 27 to 75 years with an average of 52 years (table I).

The indication for an operation was given when the complaints were undoubtful, the X-ray showed a destructive process and when conservative treatment was no longer successful.

In 72 cases (74%) we found a primary wound healing, in 12 cases (12%) a skin necrosis with only a minor delay of the healing developed. In 9 cases (9%) a dehiscence of the wound margins occurred with a subsequent complicated secondary healing. In 5 cases (5%) a wound infection developed which in 3 cases could be managed conservatively, while in 2 cases it was necessary to conduct a necrotomy in a second session (table II).

We were unable to show a direct dependence of the impaired wound healing on the base medication. To elicit that matter we revised 40 patients. All patients had received non-steroidal antiphlogistic agents. But none of the 5 patients who had undergone a base medication with Azathiopren showed signs of an impaired wound healing and only 1 of the 6 patients who had received a base medication with *D*-penicillamine suffered from impaired wound healing.

In 1 case a second resection in the area of the metatarsal II had become necessary because the metatarsal index had not primarily been preserved. At this time the patient has been operated on both sides and has no

Table III. Midterm results of arthroplasty of the forefoot by Clayton-Vainio in rheumatoid arthritis (n = 98)

Recurrent luxation	8
Hallux rigidus	1
Not performed metatarsal index	1

Table IV. Midterm results of arthroplasty of the forefoot by Clayton-Vainio in rheumatoid arthritis. Subjective improvement of patients (n = 98)

	Number	Percent
Good to excellent	84	87
Sufficient	12	11
Not sufficient	2	2

complaints. In another case a hallux rigidus developed postoperatively.

In 8 cases we saw a relapse in terms of a subluxation or even a luxation of the toes to the dorsal side. In the history of those patients there had been no gymnastics of the forefoot after the operation. However, all patients could be supplied with an orthopedic shoe which gives the patient full relief of his complaints (table III).

In 84 patients (87%) the result could be regarded as being good if not excellent. All these patients would rather undergo a second operation again which explains the high number of operations on both feet. All these patients showed, subjectively as well as objectively, a markedly improved gait.

12 patients regarded the result of their operation as being sufficient. In this group a relapse had occurred in 8 cases and in 1 case a hallux valgus had developed. These patients would only undergo a second operation under special circumstances. Two feet had to be regarded as being insufficient; both cases had been complicated by an infection. These feet can only be fully used in an orthopedic shoe (table IV).

Conclusively one has to emphasize the positive impact on both pain and gait when applying the arthroplasty by Clayton [3] and Vainio [13] which we could prove in 87% of the cases. We believe that with that technique it is not only possible to positively influence the area of the forefoot, but by means of the improved gait to reduce the mechanical stress of all the affected joints of the lower limb.

Summary

Patients with rheumatoid arthritis often developed some kind of alteration of the forefoot after a 10-year course of that disease.

If the complaints were undoubtful, the X-ray showed a destructive process and when conservative treatment was no longer successful we take the indication for the arthroplasty of the forefoot given by Clayton and Vainio.

With an average of 2 years after operation we reviewed 98 feet. In 87% the result could be regarded as being good if not excellent. 11% regarded the result of the operation as being sufficient and 2% had to be regarded as insufficient. The complications are described.

References

1 Barbier, M.: Vorfusskorrektur von dorsal oder plantar. Orthop. Praxis *5:* 533 (1976).

2 Barbier, M.; Gschwend, N.; Dybowski, R.: Die Vorfusskorrektur - Häufigkeit und Bedeutung der Zehen- und Metatarsalindices. Arch. orthop. Chir. *503:* 1 (1977).

3 Clayton, M.L.: Surgery of the forefoot in rheumatoid arthritis. Clin. Orthop. *16:* 136 (1960).

4 Fowler, A.W.: A method of forefoot reconstruction. J. Bone Jt Surg. *41B:* 507 (1959).

5 Gschwend, N.: Die operative Behandlung der chronischen Polyarthritis (Thieme, Stuttgart 1977).

6 Hoffmann, P.: An operation for severe grades of contracted or clawed toes. Am. J. orthop. Surg. *9:* 441 (1912).

7 Hohmann, G.: Fuss und Bein - Ihre Erkrankungen und deren Behandlung; 4. Aufl. (Bergmann, München 1948).

8 Kates, A.; Kassel, L.; Kay, A.: Arthroplasty of the forefoot. J. Bone Jt. Surg. *49B:* 552 (1967).

9 Short, C.; Bauer, W.; Reynolds, E.: Rheumatoid arthritis (Harvard University Press, Cambridge 1957).

10 Stamm, T.T.: Foot and ankle; in Milch: Surgery of arthritis (Williams & Wilkins, Baltimore 1964).

11 Tillmann, K.: Der rheumatische Fuss und seine Behandlung. Bücherei des Orthopäden, Band 18 (Enke, Stuttgart 1977).

12 Vahvanen, V.: Rheumatoid arthritis in the plantar joints. Acta orthop. scand. suppl. 107 (1967).

13 Vainio, K.: The rheumatoid foot. Annls Chir. Gynaec. Fenn. suppl. 1, p. 45 (1956).

Prof. Dr. H.J. Refior, MD, Orthopädische Klinik
der Medizinischen Hochschule Hannover,
Postfach 61072, D-3000 Hannover 61 (FRG)

Rheumatology, vol. 11, pp. 136–152 (Karger, Basel 1987)

Flexible Hinge Results in Implant Arthroplasty of the Great Toe

Alfred B. Swanson, Genevieve de Groot Swanson, David E. Mayhew, Ahmed Naseem Khan

Grand Rapids, Mich., USA

Resection arthroplasty of the first metatarsophalangeal joint has been commonly used for many years [1, 3, 5–7, 11]. Arthrodesis of this joint has not gained the same popularity [8]. The senior author has been interested in improving the results of arthroplasty methods at the first metatarsophalangeal joint by the use of implants as an adjunct to resection procedures [16, 17, 21]. A cobalt-chrome metal hemispherical cap with an intramedullary stem was designed in 1952, while he was an army surgeon, to replace the metatarsal head for sequelae of gunshot wounds. This procedure was used in a small number of patients. It was not considered successful because of the rigidity of the material, the shearing stress applied to the weight-bearing side of the joint, and the poor tolerance of the usually inadequate soft tissues in these cases.

A research program was instituted in 1962 to evaluate the possibilities of using a low modulus of elasticity silicone elastomer for implants for reconstruction of arthritic joints [13–22]. An intramedullary stemmed silicone implant to replace the first metatarsal head was designed in 1965; replacement of the nonweight-bearing side of the joint appeared preferable. A single stemmed silicone implant to replace the base of the proximal phalanx of the great toe was developed in 1967 to be used as an adjunct to the Keller resection arthroplasty [6]. The implant has an intramedullary stem and a slightly concave surface that articulates with the head of the metatarsal. Before the introduction of High Performance Silicone Elastomer (Dow Corning Corp., Midland, Mich.) in 1974, certain surgeons were using the finger joint implant which was made generally available in 1969 for arthroplasty of the first metatarsophalangeal joint [9]. Following the introduction of High Performance Silicone Elastomer, which has a 400% greater tear propagation resistance than the previous materials, a double-stemmed flexible hinge implant was designed in 1974 to be used as an adjunct to a Mayo-type resection arthroplasty [7]. The proximal stem of the implant fits into the intramedullary canal of the first metatarsal and the distal stem into the proximal phalanx. The flexural concavity of the implant is placed dorsally to allow a greater range of dorsiflexion of the toe.

Load Distributing Flexible Hinge

Double-stemmed flexible hinge toe implant was based on that of the well-proven flexible hinge finger joint implant with its load-distributing advantages [14–22]. The shape of this implant was developed through laboratory testing using a specially designed test machine that flexed the implant to 90° at a rate of 1,000 times a minute (fig. 1). The present implant has been flex-tested without failure more than 200 million times. The distribution of the material allows flexion to occur at the mid-section at the same time as providing both vertical and lateral stability of the flexible hinge. The mid-section has been made thicker and wider to meet the anatomic and physiologic requirements of the first metatarsophalangeal joint. This implant potentially offers better stability for maintenance of alignment and appears to be a good adjunct in reconstruction of the severely arthritic and deformed first metatarsophalangeal joint.

Concepts

The double-stemmed toe implant acts as a space filler to maintain the joint space and provide improved stability through the capsuloligamentous system that develops around the implant [14]. The use of flexible implants helps prevent joint space narrowing, allows pain-free mobility of the joint, and facilitates a normal gait pattern by the increased flexion power of the great toe during takeoff. The cosmetic appearance of the foot is improved by preserving the length and alignment of the great toe. The range of useful motion is increased because of the reduced postoperative fixation and greater joint space. Because the cap-

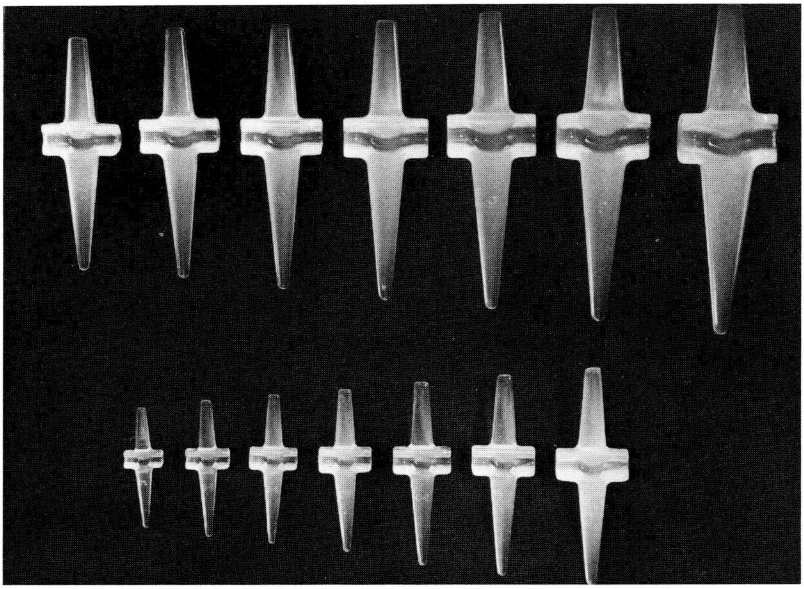

Fig. 1. The flexible hinge implant for the great toe has been designed in seven anatomic sizes. The lateral toe implants are also in seven sizes.

sule and ligaments can be reconstructed around these implants, a better and more durable correction of hallux valgus and rotational deformities can be obtained [2, 4, 9, 11, 12, 16, 17, 21, 23].

The use of implant arthroplasty for arthritic conditions of the first metatarsophalangeal joint has been a useful and rewarding procedure for our patients. The single stemmed implant is our preferred method for the treatment of hallux rigidus in younger patients who have a good metatarsal head. We now prefer the double-stemmed flexible hinge implant for severe cases of hallux rigidus or the arthritic hallux valgus and for correction of more severe deformities with destruction of both sides of the first metatarsophalangeal joint. It has found its best use in the rheumatoid arthritic foot and in the severe arthritic hallux valgus feet of the elderly patient. Proper correction of deformities must be obtained through precise release, reconstruction and balance of the soft tissues and adequate postoperative care.

A detailed review of the methods and results of single- and double-stemmed implant arthroplasty of the great toe was presented in 1977

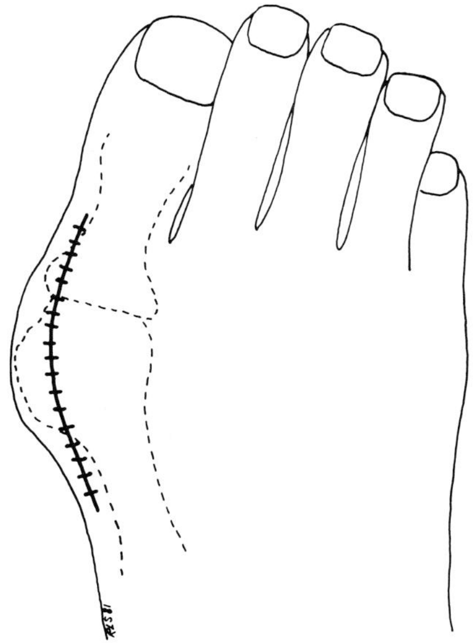

Fig. 2. A dorsomedial, slightly curved longitudinal incision is used.

[21]. The present study will emphasize the long-term results, complications and durability of the flexible hinge double-stemmed implant arthroplasty.

Methods and Materials

Double-Stemmed Flexible Hinge Toe Implant Arthroplasty

Indications. The general prerequisites of any implant arthroplasty must be respected: good condition of the patient with adequate neurovascular status and skin coverage, the possibility of a functional musculotendinous system, adequate bone stock to receive the implant, availability of postoperative therapy, and a cooperative patient.

A double-stemmed flexible hinge can be used as an adjunct to resection arthroplasty of the first metatarsophalangeal joint in the following situations: (1) In rheumatoid arthritis with hallux valgus deformity, lateral toes involvement, radiographic evidence of erosion, cyst formation and narrowing of the joint space and contractural deformities. (2) In severe senile hallux valgus deformity, care must be taken to preserve part of the head to prevent shift of weight bearing to the second toe. This procedure is also

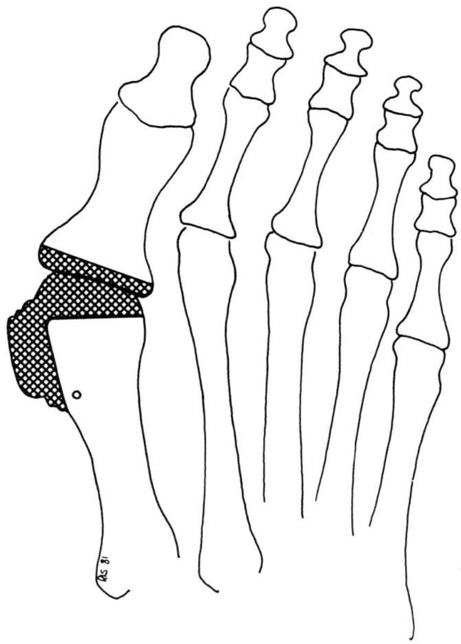

Fig. 3. The metatarsal head is excised distal to the metaphyseal flare at the largest diameter of the head with a 10° valgus angle. A portion of the base of the proximal phalanx is removed to provide a wider joint space.

recommended for hallux rigidus in the older patient. (3) In cases of moderate to severe hallux valgus deformity secondary to degenerative or posttraumatic arthritis. (4) For revision of previous procedures when there is evidence of bony destruction involving both sides of the joint and for revision procedures of failed single-stem implant arthroplasty.

Surgical Procedure. The joint is exposed through a slightly curved, longitudinal skin incision made over the dorsomedial aspect of the first metatarsophalangeal joint (fig. 2). Additional longitudinal incisions are used for reconstruction of the lateral toes as indicated. The small dorsal sensory nerves and veins in the area are avoided. The fascia and medial capsule of the joint are incised medial to the extensor hallucis longus tendon to prepare a capsuloligamentous flap for later closure and correction of the deviation deformity. This flap is usually proximally based. If the anatomical attachments appear weakened these can be reinforced with a suture through the bone, either proximally or distally. If a bursa is present, it is excised. The metatarsophalangeal joint is opened by flexing the toe and incising the dorsal capsular reflections. The capsular attachments to the neck of the metatarsal contain an important vascular supply to the bone and must be protected.

The head of the first metatarsal is excised distal to the metaphyseal flare at the largest diameter of the metatarsal head with a sagittal saw in 10° valgus to conform to normal valgus (fig. 3). The intramedullary canal is shaped in a rectangular fashion with an

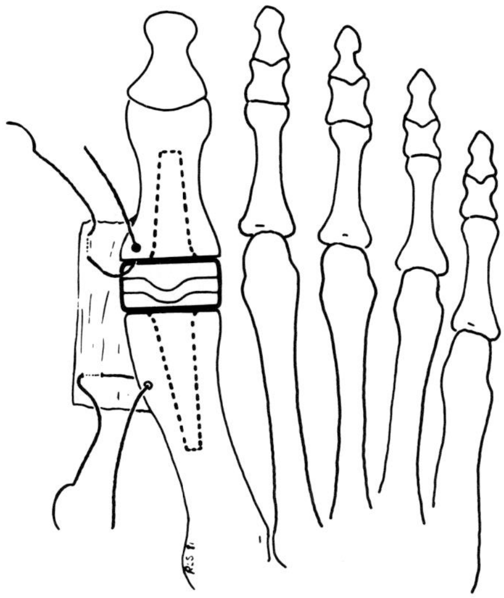

Fig. 4. The medial capsuloligamentous flap is attached to bone either distally or proximally or both.

air drill, broach or curette to accept the implant stem. A portion of the base of the proximal phalanx is removed to provide a wider joint space. Bone edges are carefully smoothened. When the lateral metatarsal heads are not resected, it is important to retain a portion of the first metatarsal head to avoid shifting of the weight bearing to the second metatarsal head. In these cases, to obtain the necessary joint space, additional bone is removed from the base of the proximal phalanx. A 0.5-mm drill hole is made in the medial portion of the metatarsal and proximal phalanx neck and 3–0 Dacron sutures are passed through these holes in preparation for capsular closure. A sizing set is available to help select the proper implant size.

The proximal (longer) stem of the implant is inserted in the intramedullary canal of the first metatarsal with the flexural concavity placed dorsally; the toe is then flexed and the distal (shorter) stem is inserted into the proximal phalanx. The proper size implant is determined by the size of the remaining metatarsal and intramedullary canal. The distal stem must not abut the end of the intramedullary canal and should be shortened as necessary. Other reshaping of the implant should be avoided.

The surgical details of the procedure and attention to the complete release of contractures, realignment of the toe ray and correction of deformities of the lateral toes are of great importance to obtain the desired results. The extensor hallucis longus is lengthened in a manner similar to a Z-plasty in cases that present a moderate to severe valgus angle and/or claw toe deformity. The tendons are sutured together with 5–0 Dexon, inverting the knots. The adductor tendon, the lateral capsule and the short flexor and extensor tendons should be released when generating deforming forces. If the intermetatarsal angle is greater than 15°, an osteotomy at the base of the first metatarsal should be considered [4, 20]. The correction of deformities and range of motion obtained at surgery will usually be that obtained in the postoperative period. In milder cases of claw toe deformity, the interphalangeal joint can be pinned with a Kirschner wire for 3–4 weeks. In cases of moderate to severe claw deformity or pronation deformity, the interphalangeal joint may require fusion. In cases of severe hallux valgus deformity, the correct alignment can be maintained in the early postoperative period by placing a 0.045-inch Kirschner wire across the toe ray in the intramedullary canals dorsal to the implant. With the implant in position, the wire is inserted in a retrograde fashion first through the intramedullary canals of the proximal and distal phalanges and then through the first metatarsal. The end of the wire extrudes 1 cm from the toe and is removed after 10 days.

With the toe held in proper longitudinal and rotational alignment, the medial fascial-capsular flap is firmly sutured proximally and distally with the previously passed Dacron sutures, burying the knots (fig. 4). The aponeurosis of the long extensor tendon, which may be released on its lateral aspect, is sutured to the medial capsule with 4–0 Dexon sutures and a buried knot technique. The long extensor tendon must be centralized with the appropriate tightness.

The skin incision is closed and small drains are placed in the wound. A voluminous conforming foot dressing is applied. Dressings are placed longitudinally to avoid circulatory compression. Cotton or Dacron batting is used for padding. A longitudinal splint such as a tongue blade, may be incorporated in the medial aspect of the dressing to support the toe in position. A posterior molded plaster splint and a conforming bandage are then applied. The foot is elevated with the patient at bed rest for 2–5 days to decrease postoperative swelling.

Postoperative Care. After 3–5 days the initial dressing is removed and a dynamic splint (US Manufacturing, Pasadena, Calif.) is applied to maintain the alignment of the toe while allowing early and active flexion-extension exercises (fig. 5). An exercise program is carefully prescribed. The dynamic splint is either attached to a cast, or is of the removable type. It is worn continuously for 3–4 weeks and then used as a night splint for approximately 3–6 weeks. The patient may walk on his heel or on a wooden-soled shoe in a week. The use of a 0.5-inch thick foam rubber inner sole extending to the distal metatarsal level is important to allow flexion exercises. Exercises over a step or other solid objects are prescribed to encourage flexion. Guarded weight bearing is allowed 3 weeks postoperatively. Appropriate nonconstrictive shoe wear is prescribed. It is most important to provide proper care of Kirschner wires extending through the skin by avoiding their extraneous movement and giving the patient adequate instructions to keep clean and dry feet. Any type of abusive foot use should be avoided postoperatively.

Patient Evaluation Method. Clinical evaluations included the patient's pain relief, shoe tolerance, walking ability, gait pattern, range of motion, toe position, and subjective satisfaction. Passive range of motion was measured as approximately 2 pounds of force were applied in both flexion and extension. Active range of motion was also noted with the patient standing with the forefoot projecting off a stool. The active range of mo-

---

Fig. 5. Postoperative splinting: *a* Dynamic splint used to allow early active flexion and extension exercises and guide the orientation of the reconstructed capsuloligamentous system. *b* The wooden-soled shoe is fitted with a 0.5-inch thick foam rubber inner sole extending to the distal metatarsal level to allow flexion exercises. *c* The dynamic toe splint worn with the wooden-soled shoe allows early weight bearing.

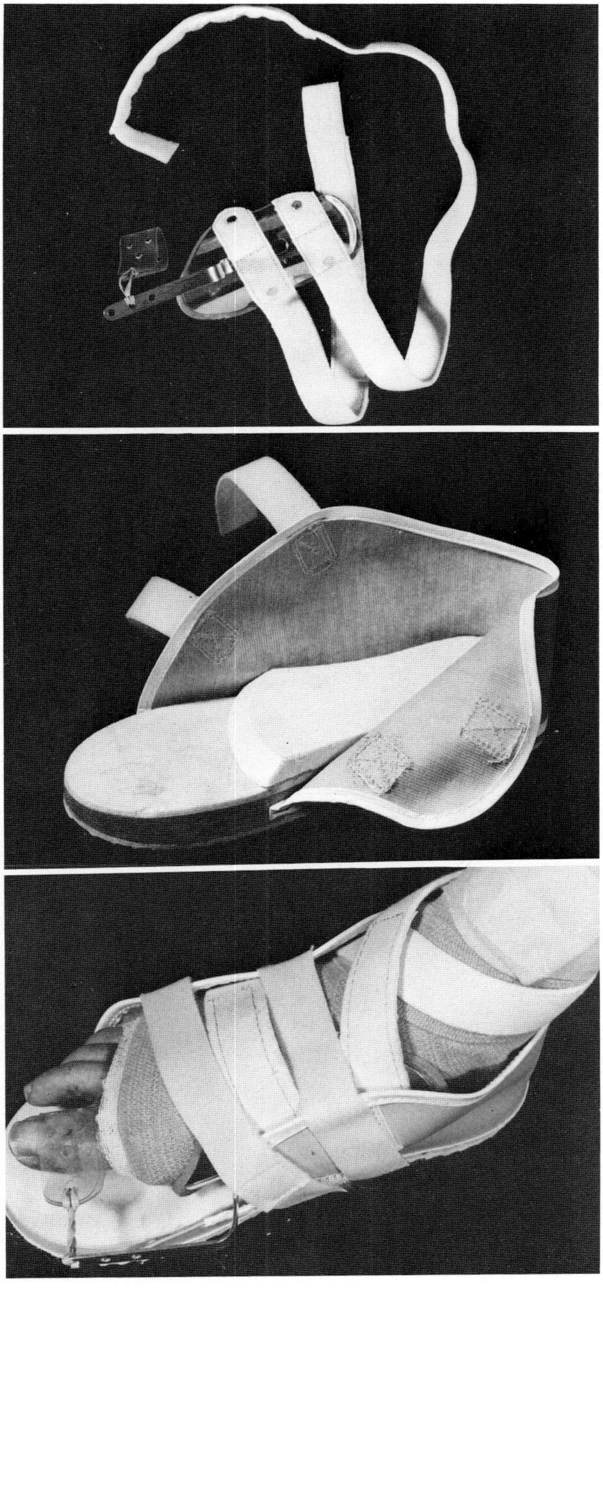

a

b

c

tion was noted to be approximately 5° less than the passive range of motion in flexion and 10° less than the passive extension. The roentgenographic joint evaluation included measurement of the metatarsophalangeal angle, evaluation of the width of the joint space, presence of erosions, cysts, and osteophyte formation. The presence of bone production, bone resorption and the status of the implant were assessed.

Results

A flexible hinge implant has been used in our clinic to reconstruct the first metatarsophalangeal joint since 1974. Patients who had a minimum of 2 years follow-up were studied to determine the long-term results. A retrospective review of all available office and research charts, specially designed foot evaluation forms, and all available preoperative and postoperative roentgenograms was carried out and included 216 patients. There were 87 bilateral cases and 8 replacement procedures for a total of 311 surgical procedures with a hinged implant. The patients' ages ranged from 16 to 75 years of age for an average of 55 years. There were 184 females and 32 males. The follow-up ranged from 28 to 129 months for an average of 77 months. The diagnoses included rheumatoid arthritis (249 toes), degenerative or osteoarthritic hallux valgus (48 toes), and hallux rigidus (6 toes). The rheumatoid cases included 234 initial procedures and 15 revisions for failure of a single stem implant arthroplasty.

A group of 31 cases with a minimum of 3 years follow-up and available preoperative, early postoperative (6 months to 1 year) and late postoperative radiograms (3–10.5 years) and clinical evaluation was separately evaluated to determine the long-term maintenance of the quality of results. This included freedom of pain, motion, toe alignment, progressive disease or late complications. The average follow-up for this separate group of patients was 92 months.

Range of Motion

A pain-free functional range of motion was obtained in the great majority of cases (table I). Compared to the preoperative arc of motion, the greatest improvement, as expected, was noted in cases of hallux rigidus who averaged 28° of arc motion preoperatively and 43° postoperatively. A comparison of the early (6–12 months) and late results (3–10.5 years) of a group of 31 cases with an average follow-up of 92 months showed a late slight decrease of movement although a func-

Table I. Great toe flexible hinge implant arthroplasty: 28–129 months follow-up (average 77 months)

Diagnosis	Number of joints	Preop. flex.	Preop. ext.	Postop. flex.	Postop. ext.	Hallux valgus, angle preop.	Hallux valgus, angle postop.
Rheumatoid arthritis	249[a]	8°	37°	7°	39°	43°	22°
Hallux valgus	48	13°	36°	13°	38°	45°	19°
Hallux rigidus	6	0°	28°	10°	33°	20°	18°
Total or average	303	9°	37°	8°	39°	42°	21°

[a] Includes 15 revisions of single-stem implant arthroplasty.

Table II. Great toe flexible hinge implant arthroplasty: early and late motion for 31 joints (92 months average follow-up)

Diagnosis	Number of joints	Preop. degrees flex.	Preop. degrees ext.	Postop. degrees early 6–12 months flex.	Postop. degrees early 6–12 months ext.	Postop. degrees late 3–10 years flex.	Postop. degrees late 3–10 years ext.
Rheumatoid arthritis	20	7	37	10	41	6	38
Hallux valgus	7	12	36	11	43	12	39
Hallux rigidus	3	0	28	11	36	10	34
Sequelae of failed reconstruction	1	0	0	9	40	10	37
Total or average	31	7	35	10	41	8	38

tional range of motion was maintained (table II). The greatest decrease in the late arc of motion was noted in the rheumatoid cases with a loss of 7° as compared to a loss of 3° in the other categories.

Hallux Valgus Angle

The hallux valgus angle was corrected to an average of 21° in 303 cases of great toe flexible hinge implant arthroplasty after an average of 77 months follow-up (table I). A comparison of the early and late re-

Table III. Great toe flexible hinge implant arthroplasty: early and late hallux valgus angle for 31 joints (92 months average follow-up)

Diagnosis	Number of joints	Hallux valgus angle		
		preop. degrees	postop. degrees	
			early range 6 months to 1 year	late range 3–10.5 years
Rheumatoid arthritis	20	42	20	23
Hallux rigidus	3	20	9	18
Hallux valgus	7	44	16	21
Sequelae of failed reconstruction	1	15	0	10
Total or average	32	39	17	22

sults in a group of 31 patients with an average 92 months follow-up showed that the best initial correction was obtained for hallux rigidus deformities (table III). Although there was an average increase of 5° in the late hallux valgus angle as compared to the early postoperative average angle, the long-term correction to 22° remained clinically cosmetic and functional.

Pain and Function

All patients had mild to severe pain, gait problems and loss of cosmesis before surgery. Postoperatively, no patients complained of pain, and had improved function and cosmesis through improved gait patterns, mobility and toe length and alignment.

Complications

Wound Complications. Wound problems should be considered in three separate categories: (1) early infections occurring within 6 weeks after surgery; (2) late skin breakdowns occurring one year or more after normal wound healing has taken place. These can be related to improper shoe fit, abusive foot use or breakdown of an overlying rheumatoid nodule; and (3) delayed healing with stabilization of the wound 4–9 weeks after surgery.

In our series of 303 cases, there were 3 early postoperative infections with a skin breakdown and exposure of the implant that could not be salvaged by conservative measures. The implant was removed and not replaced in all 3 cases. A late skin breakdown occurred in 2 patients; one at 2 years and one at 3 years after surgery. One patient had an overlying rheumatoid nodule that became ulcerated. In both cases the implant was removed and not replaced. Delayed wound healing that responded well to conservative measures of rest and antibiotic therapy was noted in 9 of 303 operated feet.

Synovitis. A reactive synovitis was noted in 4 of the 303 cases with evidence of some degree of translucency around at least one of the implant stems on the radiograms. In 3 of these cases a revision procedure was carried out. In 2 of these cases there was an associated implant fracture; the implant was removed and replaced at 29 months and 48 months after each initial procedure. In one case there was associated bony overgrowth; abrasion of the implant midsection and reactive synovitis were noted at the time of implant removal and replacement 34 months after the initial procedure. A synovectomy was also carried out in these cases. Following the revision procedure, favorable bone remodeling occurred. The fourth case is currently under clinical observation.

Angulation Deformity. A recurrent valgus angle to greater than 30° was noted in 3 of the 303 cases. In 2 cases a soft tissue revision procedure to realign the capsuloligamentous structures was carried out along with implant removal and replacement. A secondary lengthening of the extensor hallux longus was carried out in one case. The implant was found to be intact in both cases. The third case refused a revision procedure. In 7 cases, a recurrence of valgus deformity of less than 30° was noted. However, these patients did not present pain or discomfort with shoe wear and did not require a secondary procedure.

A surgical overcorrection to a mild varus angle was noted in 2 cases. Due to the lack of clinical discomfort no revision surgery was required.

A mild extension deformity that did not require a revision procedure was noted in 5 cases. Earlier in our surgical experience the importance of proper balance of the extensor/flexor mechanism had been recognized and was rewarded with improved results.

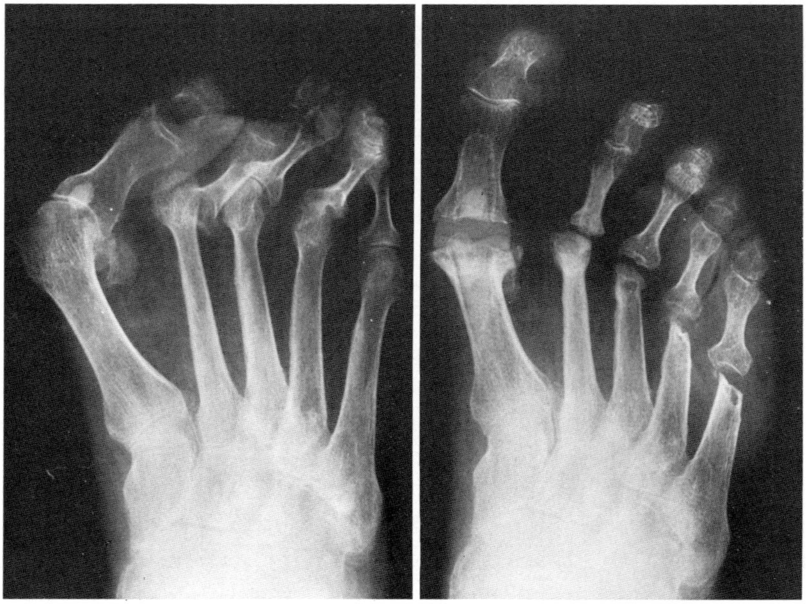

a b

Fig. 6. a Preoperative radiogram showing typical rheumatoid arthritis deformities with involvement of the great toe and lateral toes. *b* Radiogram 3 years following flexible hinge implant resection arthroplasty of the great toe and resection arthroplasty of the MTP joints of the lateral toes. Note good correction of deformities, implant tolerance as demonstrated by apposite of new bone around the stems.

Implant Fractures. There were 6 implant fractures noted in 303 flexible hinge implant arthroplasty cases. In 4 cases the implant was removed and replaced. Associated reactive synovitis was present in 2 of these cases. In 1 case who had a late skin breakdown, the implant was removed and not replaced. In the last case the implant fracture was noted on radiograms and a revision procedure has not been carried out to date.

Bone Production. The bone remodeling phenomena that occur around silicone flexible hinges had been previously reported for a series of 120 metacarpophalangeal joints [19]. Similar findings were obtained for the first metatarsophalangeal joint flexible hinge implant arthroplasty. A favorable bone remodeling was demonstrated in most cases by apposition of new bone around the intramedullary stems and thickening of the cortical bone at the resected bone ends in contact with the implant midsection (fig. 6). 'Lipping' of the bone ends is a sign of periosteal bone overproduction at the cut end of the bones. A mild degree of 'lipping' which does not interfere with the joint space does not affect the quality of results. This is common and was noted in 13 of our 31 cases of long-term follow-up. A severe degree of bone overgrowth that required surgical revision was noted in 2 of our 303 cases. In both cases there was a loss of motion. In one case there were signs of implant abrasion and reactive synovitis.

Bone Absorption. Bone absorption must be a critical point in evaluating the long-term result of joint implants. It is usually a manifestation of an inflammatory or disease process. Bone absorption around the intramedullary stem was seen in 4 of our cases in association with reactive synovitis and implant fracture or abrasion as previously described. Cystic and erosive changes were very rare and were noted in 2 cases who had large cysts of the metatarsal head preoperatively.

Revision Procedures

There were a total of 13 revision procedures in 303 cases. In 5 cases the implant was removed and not replaced due to infection (3), or late wound breakdown (2), as previously described. Conversion to a simple resection arthroplasty provided satisfactory clinical and functional results in these cases due to the establishment of a capsuloligamentous system during the early healing period. In 8 cases the implant was removed and replaced for reasons previously explained: implant fracture (2), recurrent valgus (2), synovitis with implant fracture (2), synovitis with bone overgrowth and implant abrasion (1), and isolated bone overgrowth (1). A satisfactory clinical and functional result followed these simple revision procedures.

Discussion

The review of 303 cases of flexible implant resection arthroplasty of the great toe with an average 77 months follow-up and of a series of 31 cases with both early (6–12 months) and late (3–10.5 years) results averaging 92 months follow-up has been carried out. The use of a double-stemmed implant for the rheumatoid foot and in cases of moderate to severe hallux valgus deformity and destruction of both sides of the joint has provided excellent long-term pain relief with functional mobility, alignment and stability. A comparison of early and late results has demonstrated that a slight loss of correction occurs in the late follow-up without compromising the functional quality of the results.

Spontaneous, early postoperative infections should not occur unless there is a break in the operative technique or method of implant sterilization. In our 3 cases of early postoperative infection we found that the skin breakdown was initiated by a superficially placed suture in patients with poor skin quality. The importance of the surgical technique, use of proper suture material, inversion of surgical knots, meticulous pin care, if used, and adequate shoe prescription must be stressed to avoid these complications, especially in the often steroid-dependent rheumatoid patients.

A fracture of the flexible hinge implant occurred in 6 of 303 cases. We feel that tearing of the flexible hinge is most often initiated by pinching or cutting of the implant by sharp bone edges across a tight subluxating joint or a joint that has become loosened through recurrent synovitis. In an effort to improve the durability of the implant, a research project was initiated in 1976 to develop an acceptable shielding device to protect the flexible hinge midsection from excessive wear. Laboratory, animal and human clinical studies using eight different materials with or without bony ingrowth have shown that a titanium press-fit bone liner (grommet) can effectively protect the flexible hinge implants without interfering with the favorable bone response usually presented at the implant/bone interface [18]. The early results appear promising in both implant protection, and maintenance of the shape of the cut bone ends.

Cystic or erosive changes may be the continued manifestation of the arthritic process. Inflammatory manifestations around the implant can usually be identified on radiologic examination by the presence of an 'intramedullary sign'. Normally a bony shell is formed intimately to the implant stems. If this line is missing or if there is widening of the space between the implant and the cortical line, an inflammatory process should be suspected. The implant may aggravate this process if excessive wear particles are formed. A reactive synovitis was found on microscopic examination of pathology specimens of 3 cases of implant removal and replacement. In 2 cases there was an implant fracture and in 1 case the implant was abraded from a bony overgrowth. The microscopic evaluation showed the presence of a foreign body giant cell reaction in the presence of silicone particles without necrosis or malignant changes. Intracellular ovoid particles varying from 3 to 13 μm in size which tended to clump together were observed. A few extracellular particles were seen and these tended to be singular and of smaller size. We feel that silicone particles can participate in a foreign body giant cell reaction and reactive synovitis as seen with many other inert materials [10, 20]. This has been shown not to be an immune type reaction as immune competent cells including antibody-producing plasma cells have been noticeably scarce in the material examined. If there is evidence of persistent synovitis with bone change, the implant should be removed and simple resection arthroplasty results. The implant can also be replaced or an arthrodesis with a bone graft can be considered. Recently the use of a metal bone shielding (grommet) device appears to effectively protect the implant from the cutting action of sharp bone edges and thereby decrease wear particles.

This review of flexible hinge implant arthroplasty has demonstrated that the great majority of patients have benefited from improved cosmesis, function and freedom of pain. It is our opinion that this procedure can be a useful adjunct to resection arthroplasty of the arthritic first metatarsophalangeal joint if proper indications, surgical and postoperative measures are carried out.

References

1 Clayton, M.L.: Surgery of the forefoot in rheumatoid arthritis. J. Bone Jt Surg. *42A:* 523 (1960).
2 Cracchiolo, A.; Swanson, A.B.; Swanson, G. de Groot: The arthritic great toe metatarsophalangeal joint. A review of flexible silicone implant arthroplasty from two medical centers. Clin. Orthop. *157:* 64–69 (1981).
3 Giannestras, N.J.: Foot disorders; 2nd ed. (Lea & Febiger, Philadelphia 1976).
4 Gould, N.: Surgery of the forepart of the foot in rheumatoid arthritis. Foot Ankle *3:* 173–180 (1982).
5 Hoffman, P.: An operation for severe grades of contracted or claw toes. Am. J. orthop. Surg. *9:* 441 (1911).
6 Keller, W.L.: Surgical treatment of bunions and hallux valgus. N.Y. med. J. *80:* 741–742 (1904).
7 Mayo, C.M.: The surgical treatment of bunions. Ann. Surg. *48:* 300 (1908).
8 McKeever, D.C.: Arthrodesis of the first metatarsophalangeal joint for hallux valgus and hallux rigidus and metatarsus primus varus. J. Bone Jt Surg. *34A:* 129 (1952).

9 Michon, J.; Delagoutte, J.P.; Jandeaux, M.: L'Arthroplastie par implants en silastic dans la cure de l'hallux valgus et des arthrites aseptiques de l'articulation metatarsophalangienne. Actual. Méd. Chir. Pied *8:* 209–214 (1973).

10 Nalbandian, R.M.; Swanson, A.B.; Maupin, B.K.: Long-term silicone implant arthroplasty. J. Am. med. Ass. *2:* 1195–1198 (1983).

11 Smith, R.W.; Wagner, F.W., Jr.: Disorders of the forefoot. Clin. Orthop. *142:* 2–3 (1979).

12 Snedden, H.E.: Implant arthroplasty in the treatment of painful bunions. Proc. 48th Annu. Meet. of the Am. Academy of Orthopaedic Surgeons, Las Vegas 1981.

13 Swanson, A.B.: Improving the end-bearing characteristics of lower extremity amputation stumps. N.Y. Univ. Inter.-Clin. Inform. Bull. *5:* 1–7 (1966).

14 Swanson, A.B.: Finger joint replacement by silicone rubber implants and the concept of implant fixation on encapsulation. Ann. rheum. Dis. *28:* suppl., pp. 47–55 (1969).

15 Swanson, A.B.: Flexible implant arthroplasty for arthritic finger joints. Rationale, technique and results of treatment. J. Bone Jt Surg. *54A:* 435–455 (1972).

16 Swanson, A.B.: Implant arthroplasty for the great toe. Clin. Orthop. *85:* 75–81 (1972).

17 Swanson, A.B.: Flexible implant resection arthroplasty in the hand and extremities (Mosby, St. Louis 1973).

18 Swanson, A.B.: A grommet bone liner for flexible implant arthroplasty. Bull. Pros. Res. Rehab. Eng. Res. Devel. *18:* 108–114 (1981).

19 Swanson, A.B.; Swanson, G. de Groot: Bone remodeling phenomena in flexible (silicone) implant arthroplasty in the hand. Long-term study. Kappa Delta Award Lecture. 49th Annu. Meet. of Orthopaedic Surgeons, New Orleans 1982. Orthop. Rev. *11:* 129–131 (1982).

20 Swanson, A.B.; Swanson, G. de Groot; Frisch, E.E.: Flexible (silicone) implant arthroplasty in the small joints of extremities. Concepts, physical and biological considerations, experimental and clinical results; in Rubin, Biomaterials in reconstructive surgery, pp. 595–623 (Mosby, St. Louis 1983).

21 Swanson, A.B.; Lumsden, R.M.; Swanson, G. de Groot: Silicone implant arthroplasty of the great toe. Clin. Orthop. *142:* 30 (1979).

22 Swanson, A.B.; Meester, W.D.; Swanson, G. de Groot ; Rangaswamy, L.; Schut, G.E.D.: Durability of silicone implants. An in vivo study. Orthop. Clin. North Am. *4:* 1097–1112 (1973).

23 Wenger, R.J.J.; Whalley, R.C.: Total replacement of the first metatarsophalangeal joint. J. Bone Jt Surg. *60B:* 88–92 (1978).

Alfred B. Swanson, MD, Blodgett Professional Building, Suite 290,
1900 Wealthy Street, SE, Grand Rapids, MI 49506 (USA)

Rheumatology, vol. 11, pp. 153–160 (Karger, Basel 1987)

Surgery of the Forefoot in Advanced Rheumatoid Arthritis

H.C. Meuli

Lindenhofspital Bern, Schweiz

In the complex foot the painful forefoot is a prime source of difficulty in walking. Therefore the forefoot deformities represent a main indication for surgical treatment. Resection arthroplasty of the metatarsophalangeal joints is a well-known procedure. It is generally accepted and most appreciated by the patients. A number of different surgical techniques has been published [1–4]. Usually the operation is performed through a dorsal or a plantar approach to the lateral four metatarsal heads. The great toe is usually approached through a dorsal or dorsomedial incision. For a long period of time we have been using these incisions in a modification of the technique described by Lelièvre [3] with satisfactory results. Since we know that incisions through the sole heal well and do not give rise to neuromata, we prefer this approach especially in the complex foot with severe forefoot deformities. Some years ago we started to use a plantar approach to all metatarsophalangeal joints including the great toe. This technique proved to be very advantageous for several reasons: only one incision is needed; an excellent view is provided; the extensor tendons are not touched and no irritation and stiffening by scar tissue has to be expected; an excision of the plantar callosities is possible, and the dermadesis allows the fat pad to be drawn back into its anatomical position. A floppy forefoot can thus be prevented.

Surgical Technique (fig. 1–12)

A lip of the plantar surface skin which is associated with callosities and ulcerations is excised. Thus an excellent approach to the four dropped lateral metatarsal heads is

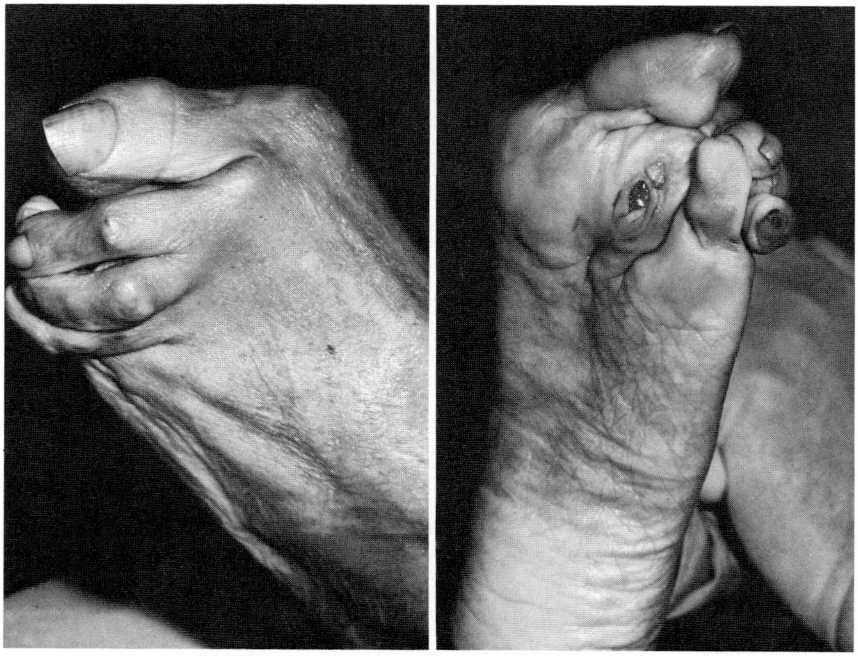

1a, b

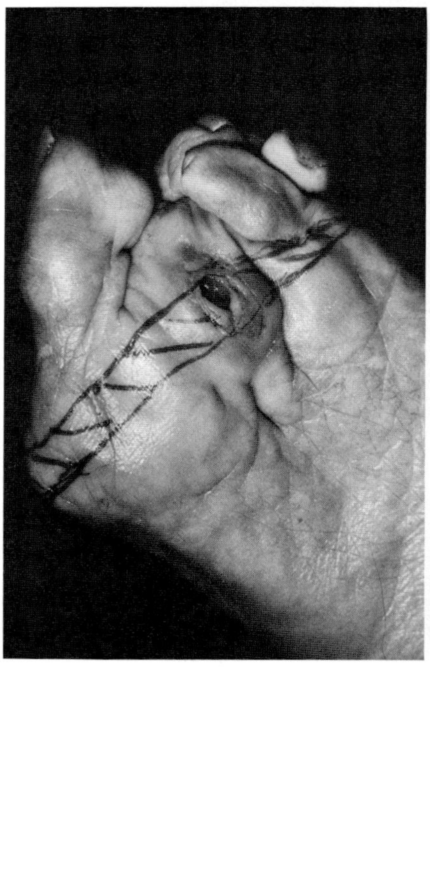

2

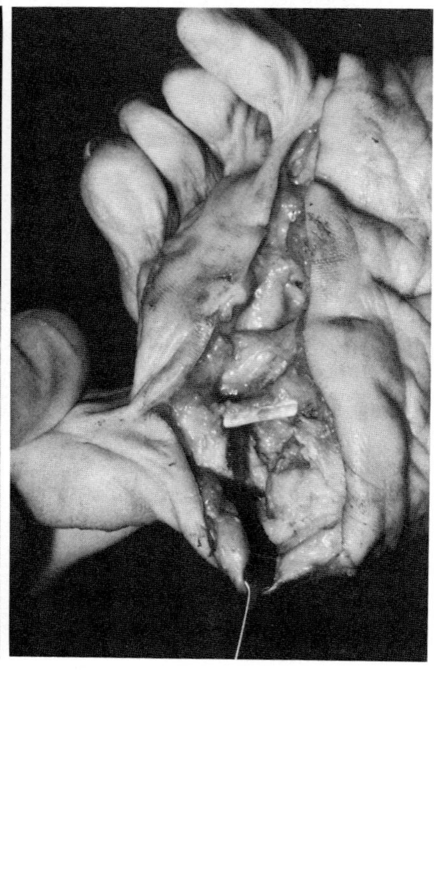

3

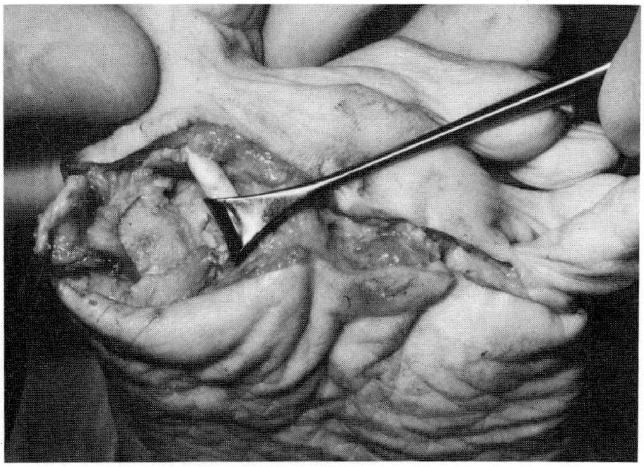

4

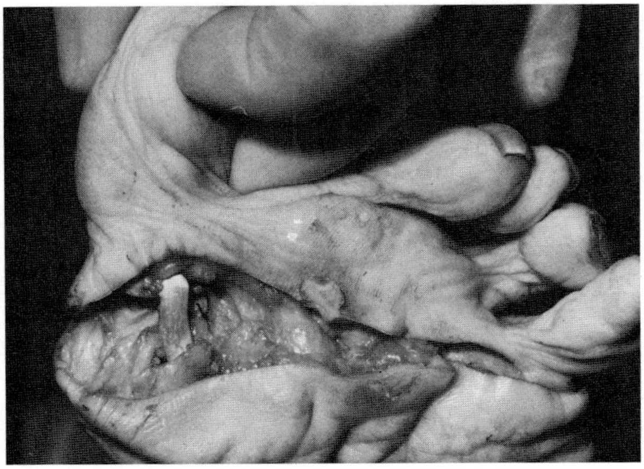

5

Fig. 4. Modelling of the metatarsal head I. Preparing of the capsular flap.

Fig. 5. Capsular flap interposed.

Fig. 1. a, b Forefoot deformity before surgery.

Fig. 2. Skin incision.

Fig. 3. Approach to the metatarsophalangeal joint I. Resection of the basis of the phalanx performed.

6 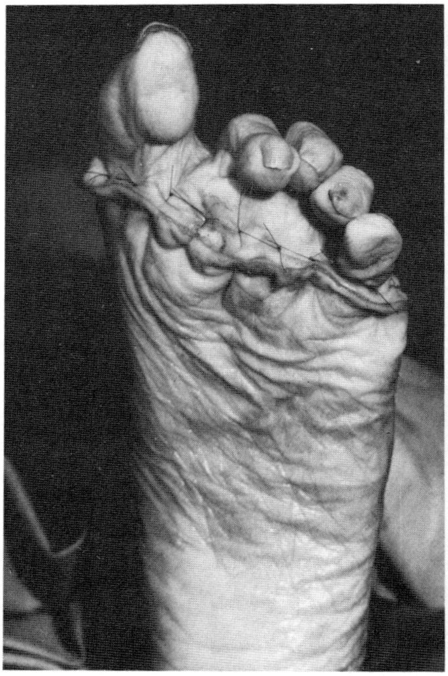

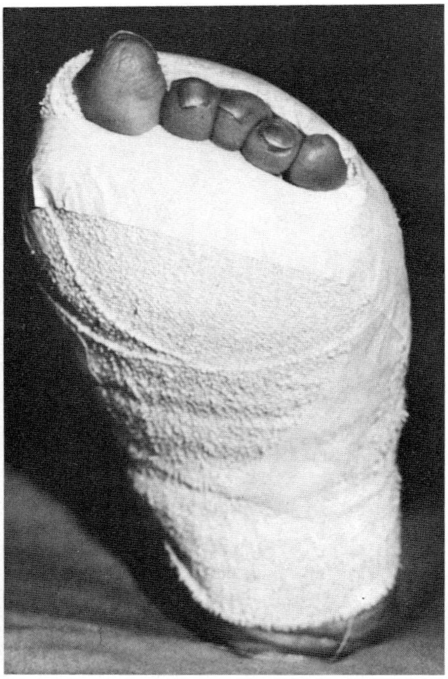 7

Fig. 6. Wound closed – dermadesis.
Fig. 7. Soft compressive dressing.
Fig. 8. a, b Two weeks postoperative.
Fig. 9. a, b Corrective elastic dressing.

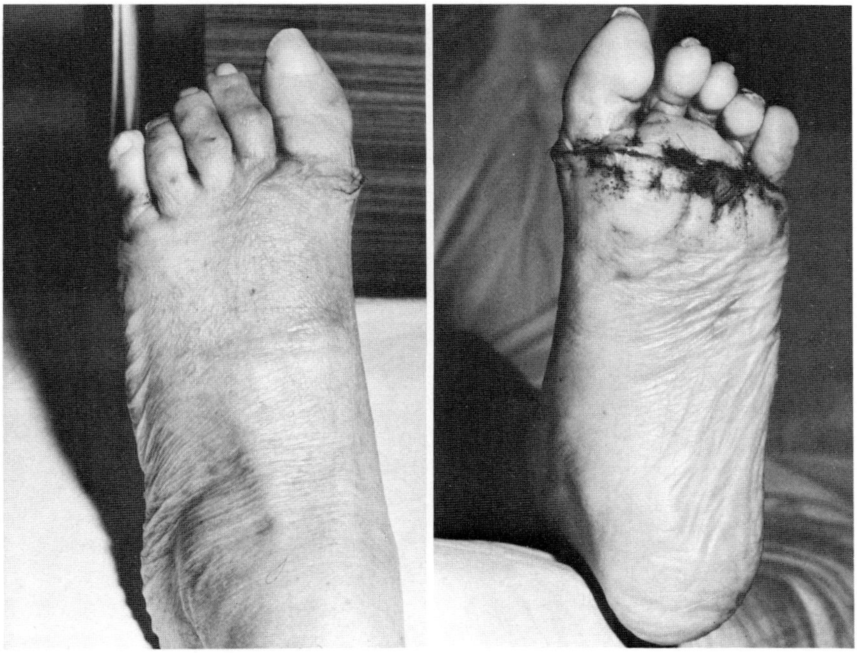

8a, b

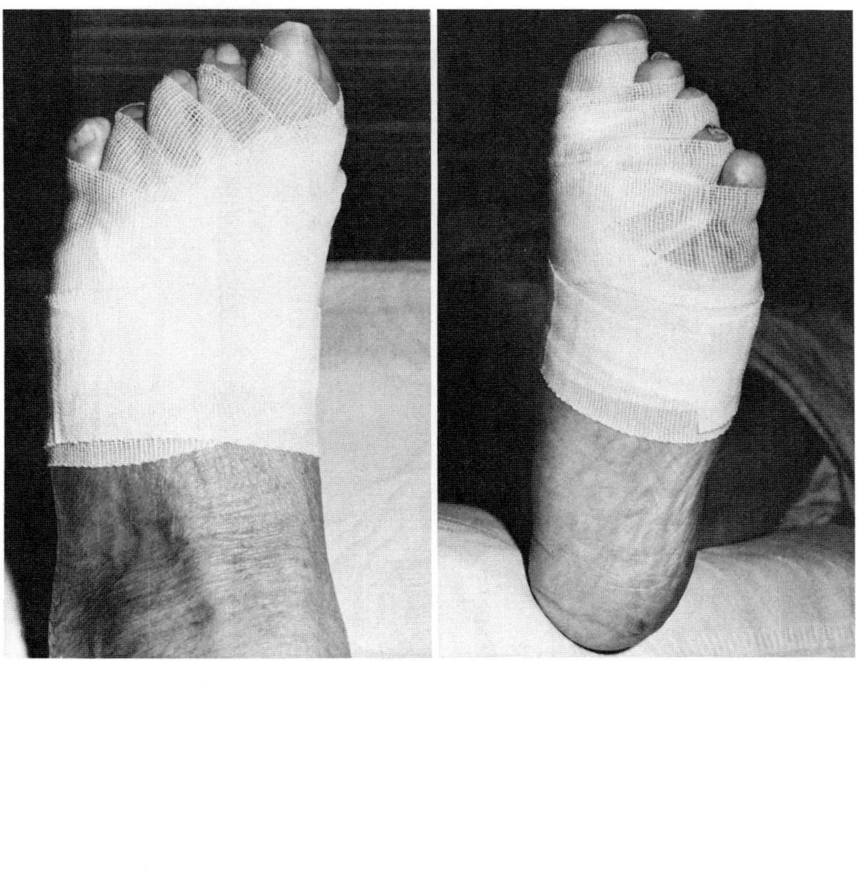

9a, b

a 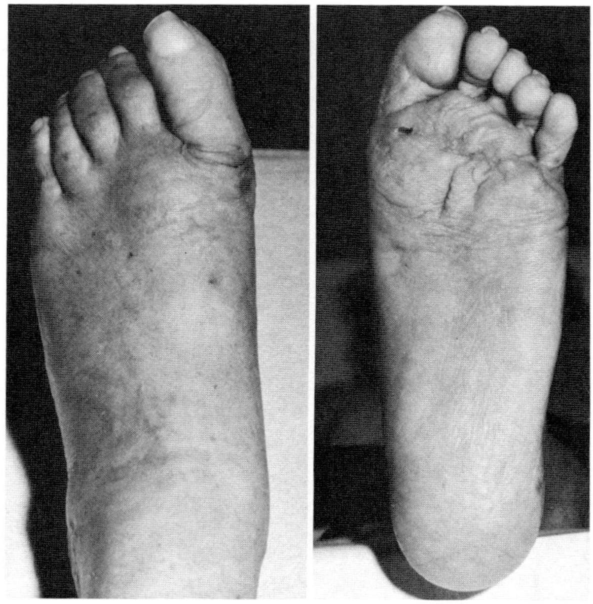 b

Fig. 10. a, b Six weeks postoperative.

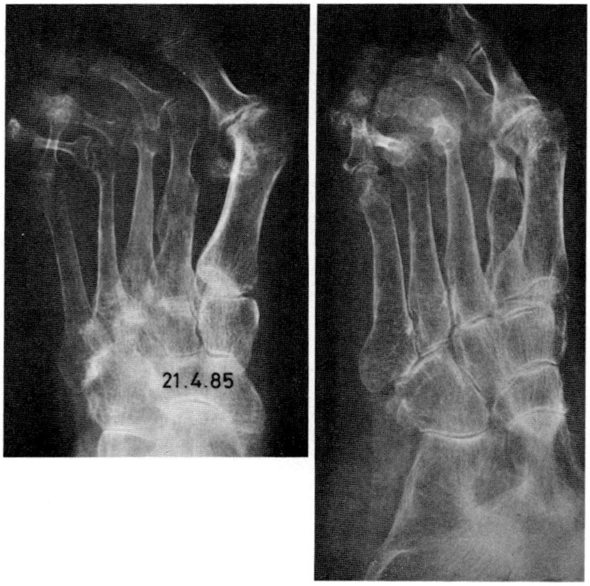

Fig. 11. X-Ray – preoperative.

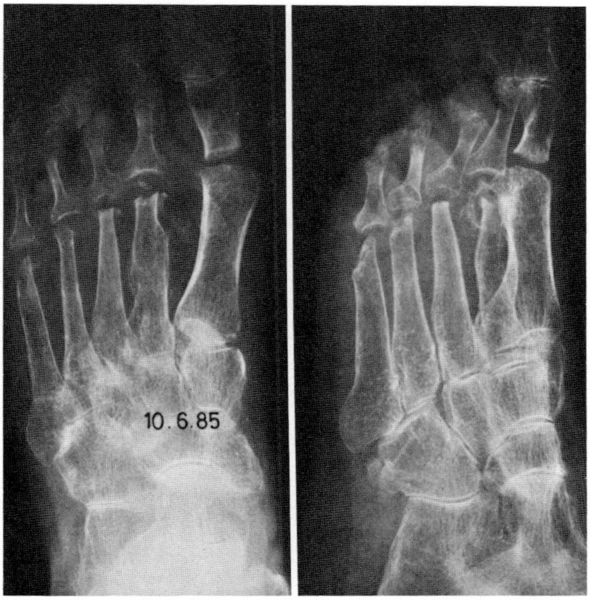

Fig. 12. X-Ray – postoperative.

achieved. The metatarsal heads II–V are resected in the usual way. Then the first metatarsophalangeal joint is approached: a proximally based capsular flap can be prepared easily because the flexor tendons are displaced laterally as well as the neurovascular bundle. The joint is opened laterally through a longitudinal incision. The extent of bone resection has to be calculated carefully – according to the measurements on the preoperative X-rays. The first metatarsal head is freed completely and molded. The capsular flap is interposed and dorsolaterally sutured over the metatarsal head. The flexor tendon is reduced with the sesamoids which usually are not removed to avoid a dysbalance of the tendons of the first toe. Thus the first metatarsal is realigned and stabilized ('cerclage fibreux') [3]. The incision is closed and the dermadesis provides an excellent correction of the deformed toes. The stability is astonishingly good and no internal or external fixation is needed.

A soft compressive dressing is applied to hold the toes in the desired position. This dressing is removed after one week. Walking with guarded weight bearing is then allowed. A corrective dressing with an elastic bandage is applied for at least 6 weeks.

This is a preliminary report. We are not in the position to present long-term results. However, the cosmetic and functional results of the first few cases are extremely satisfactory and comparable with other procedures. The technique might be recommendable in the surgical treatment of severe forefoot disorders in advanced rheumatoid arthritis.

Summary

A new technique for resection arthroplasty of the metatarsophalangeal joints, using the plantar approach to all metatarsals including the great toe is discussed. With this technique, a correction of severe deformities can be achieved. It seems to be advantageous that the extensor tendons of the great toe are not touched, such avoiding scar problems. The skin, which often is associated with plantar ulceration, is excised and by closing the skin an excellent correction of the position of the toes is achieved (dermodesis). These incisions through the sole heal astonishingly well and usually there are no problems with neuromata or deforming scar. The cosmetic and the functional results of the first few cases treated with this technique are extremely satisfactory.

References

1 Clayton, M.L.: Surgery of the forefoot in rheumatoid arthritis. Clin. Orthop. *16:* 136 (1960).
2 Gschwend, N.: Die operative Behandlung der progressiv chronischen Polyarthritis (Thieme, Stuttgart 1967).
3 Lelièvre, J.: Pathologie du pied (Masson, Paris 1952).
4 Tillmann, K.: Der rheumatische Fuss und seine Behandlung (Enke, Stuttgart 1977).

Prof. Dr. Hans-Christoph Meuli, Lindenhofspital Bern, CH-3012 Bern (Schweiz)

Rheumatology, vol. 11, pp. 161–172 (Karger, Basel 1987)

How Do Various Operative Procedures on the Forefoot Influence the Rheumatoid Foot

F.-W. Hagena, W. Bracker, T.-F. Hoffmann, B. Rosemeyer, Th. Zwingers

Staatliche Orthopädische Klinik der Ludwig-Maximilian-Universität und Biometrisches Zentrum für Therapiestudien, München, BRD

Several different operative procedures on the rheumatoid forefoot are well known [Hoffmann, 1911; Fowler, 1959; Clayton, 1960; Kates et al., 1967; Lelièvre, 1952; Lipscomb et al., 1972; Tillmann, 1973]. 50% of the rheumatoid patients suffer from problems of the forefoot [Vainio, 1956; Tillmann, 1977]. Comparative studies on different operative procedures are rare.

Materials and Methods

Between 1973 and 1983, 91 rheumatoid feet were operated on at the Staatliche Orthopädische Klinik, Munich, with arthroplasties of the MTP joints. We report here the results of a follow-up study of 46 feet in 27 patients with an average follow-up time of 6.5 years. In the meantime, 7 patients have died, 6 have moved and 14 were not traced.

Of the 46 feet, 19 were operated on bilaterally. The average age of the patients at operation was 59 years, the average time of duration of rheumatoid arthritis was 14.5 years (min. 2 years, max. 51 years).

In this study of 46 feet, 25 cases underwent the dorsal approach and 21 cases underwent the plantar approach. Four years ago we changed our operative regimen so that the patients with dorsal approach have an average time of review of 9 years and those with plantar approach are reviewed after a mean time of 3.5 years (table I). There is also a difference between the types of resection methods for the arthroplasties of the forefeet. 10 feet had only resections of the metatarsal I heads, whereas in 36 feet the base of the proximal phalanges at the hallux were removed too.

Figure 1 and table II show the distribution of the different resections at phalanges II–V. When there was a resection of the metatarsal heads, additional resections of the heads of the proximal phalanges occurred in 7 cases.

Table I. Material and times of review (1973–1983)

Number of patients	
Total	54
Reviewed	27
Number of feet	
Total	91
Reviewed	46
Unilateral	8
Bilateral	19
Time of review generally	
Minimum	2 years
Maximum	13 years
Average	6.5 years
Time of review versus approach	
Dorsal	9 years
Plantar	3.5 years
Review not possible	
Died	7
Not located	14
Moved	6
Duration of the rheumatoid disease	
Minimum	2 years
Maximum	51 years
Average	14.5 years
Age at operation	
Minimum	36 years
Maximum	75 years
Average	59.2 years

Results

In the 46 feet including the different operative procedures, we found a decrease of pain in 78% and better ability to walk in 76% of the cases in total. The cosmetic aspect was better in 20% and unchanged in 46% of the feet. In two thirds of all cases the postoperative situation showed an objective and subjective improvement (table III).

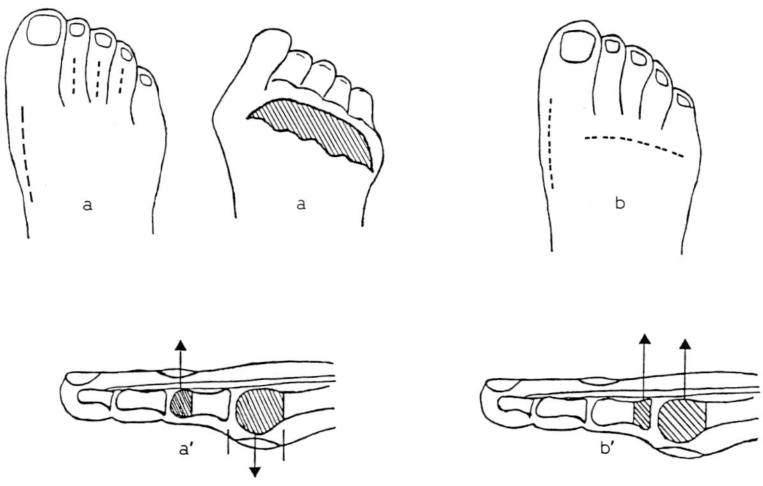

Fig. 1. Different operation procedures. a = Dorsomedial approach for the hallux, facultative dorsal incision for the resection of the proximal phalanx head; plantar approach for toes II–V; a′ = metatarsal head resection, facultative proximal phalanx head resection; b = dorsal approach for toes I–V; b′ = metatarsal head resection and proximal phalanx base resection.

Table II. Dimension of resection versus approach

Resection	Approach	
	plantar	dorsal
MTP joint I		
MTH I	5	5
MTH I + PPB I	16	20
MTP joints II–V		
MTH + PPB II–V	5	25
MTH II–V + PPH (facultative)	16 (7)	–

MTH = metatarsal head; PPB = base of the proximal phalanx; PPH = head of the proximal phalanx.

Table III. Results of 46 feet with different operative procedures

	Pain %	Ability to walk %	Cosmetic aspect %	Opinion patient/doctor %
Better	36/78	35/76	9/20	30/28
Unchanged	4/9	6/13	22/47	6/8
Worse	6/13	5/11	15/33	10/10

Table IV. Pain versus approach and resection of toes II–V

Pain	Approach		Resection	
	plantar	dorsal	MTH (+PPH)	MTH+PPB
No	10	6	6	10
Moderate	9	8	8 9	
Serious	2	11	2	11

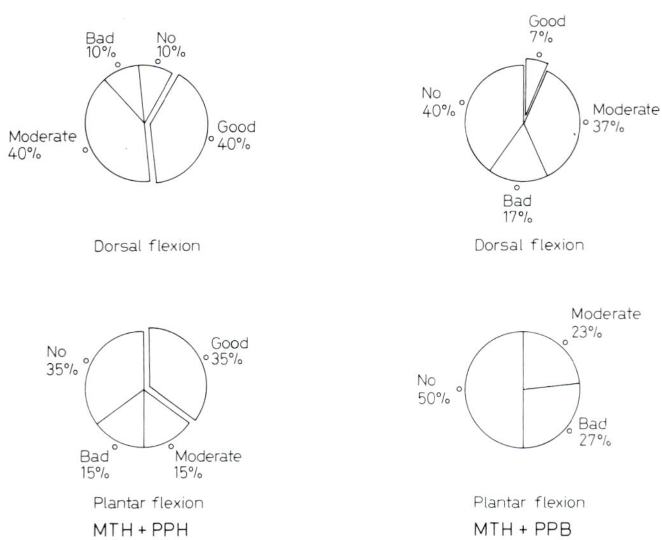

Fig. 2. ROM versus resection phalanges II–V.

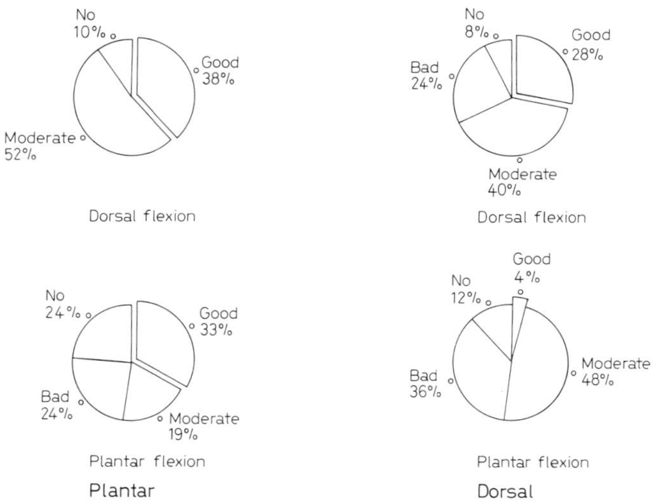

Fig. 3. ROM versus approach hallux.

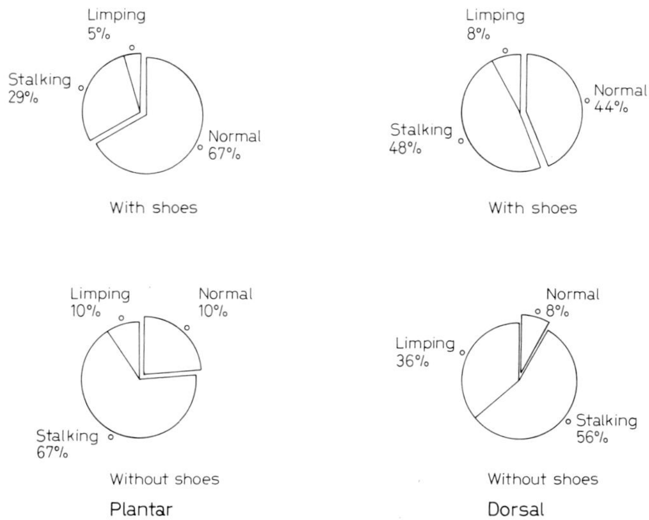

Fig. 4. Ability to walk versus approach.

Table V. Orthopedic aids versus approach and resection postoperatively

Orthopedic aids	Total	Approach		Resection	
		plantar	dorsal	MTH (+PPH)	MTH+PPB
Orthopedic shoes	24	5	19	4	20
Normal shoes	22	16	6	12	10
Total	46	21	25	16	30

Table VI. Number of feet with luxated toes (postoperatively) versus approach

Luxations	Approach		Resection	
	plantar %	dorsal %	MTH %	MTH+PPB %
No	76	32	75	40
Yes	24	68	25	60

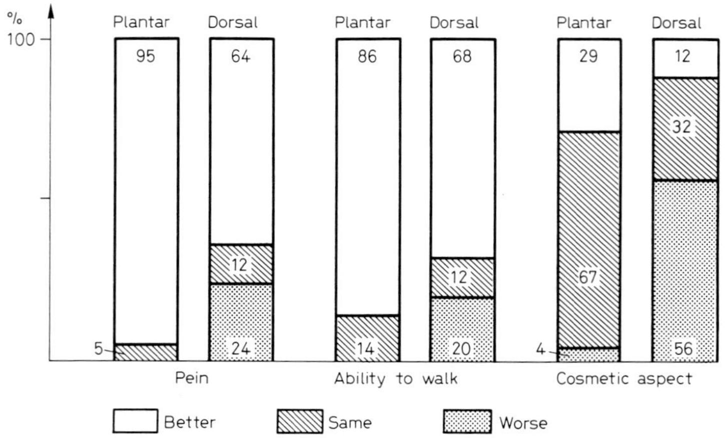

Fig. 5. Subjective estimation of the patients according to approach.

Table VII. Doctors' opinion according to approach

	Approach		Resection	
	plantar %	dorsal %	MTH %	MTH+PPB %
Good	71	20	69	33
Satisfactory	19	48	18	40
Not satisfactory	10	32	13	27

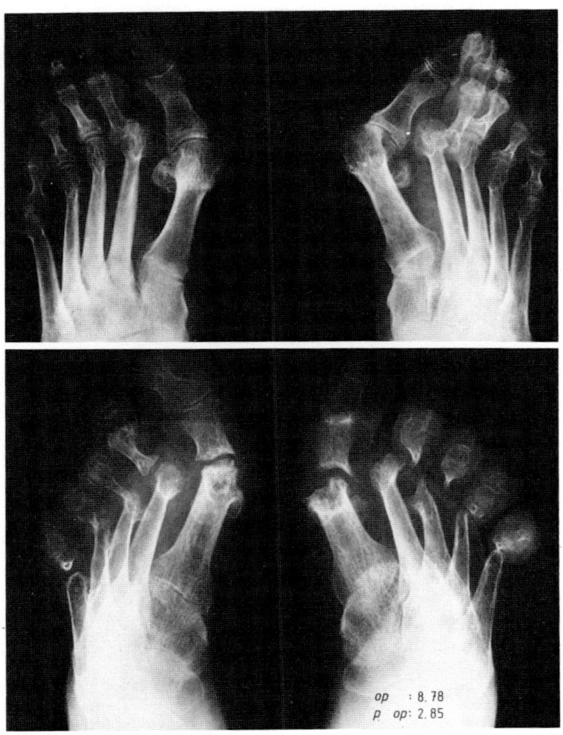

Fig. 6. Patient, 62-year-old female, 14 years RA. *a* Preoperative X-ray. *b* Postoperative X-ray, 7 years after dorsal approach, resection of metatarsal heads and bases of the proximal phalanges.

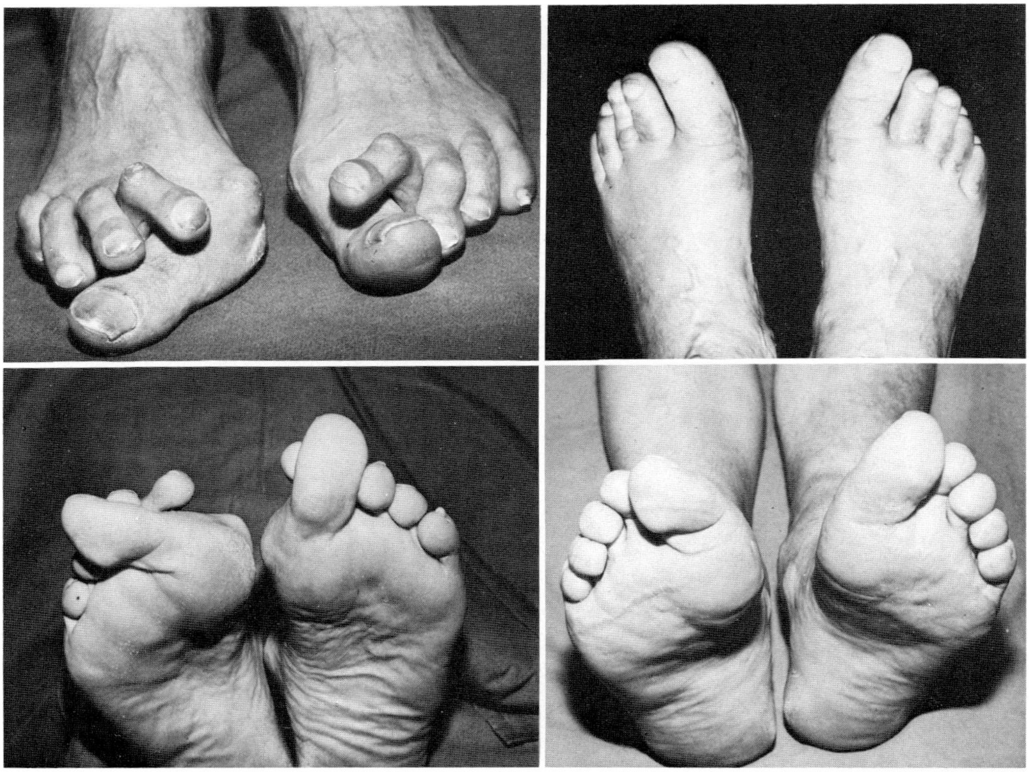

Fig. 7. Patient, 57-year-old female 16 years RA. *a–d* Clinical documentation pre- and postoperatively, 4.5 years after plantar approach, resection of the metatarsal heads and heads of proximal phalanges II and III. *e, f* Pre- and postoperative X-ray, hallux valgus deformity because of too small resection of metatarsus I. *g* Intraoperative aspect of plantar approach with resection of a bursa at MTP V.

Pain is the main indication for forefoot arthroplasties. 6 of 25 cases with dorsal approach were pain-free whereas 10 of 21 feet with plantar approach were pain-free. Comparing the different patients we can also see that those feet with resections of the metatarsal heads and facultative resection of the heads of the proximal phalanges in 50% have no pain. Only 20% of those operated on by the technique of Clayton-Vainio are as successful as this (table IV).

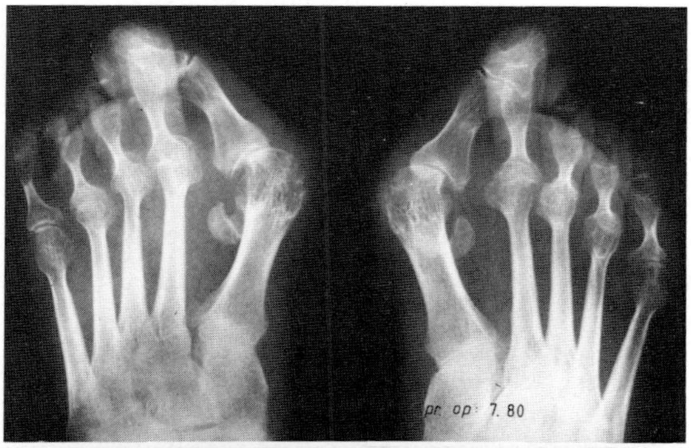

7, e

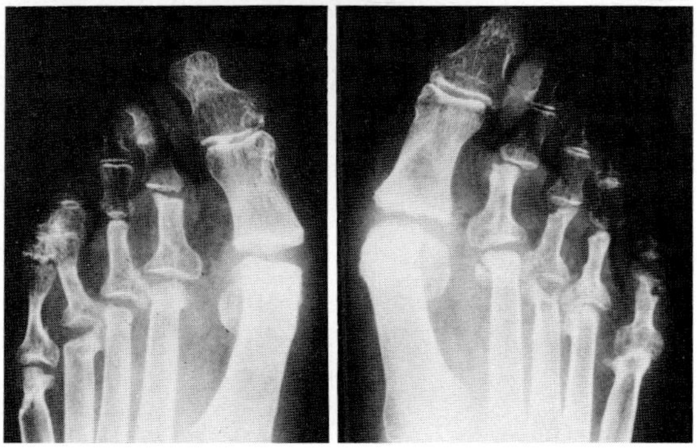

f

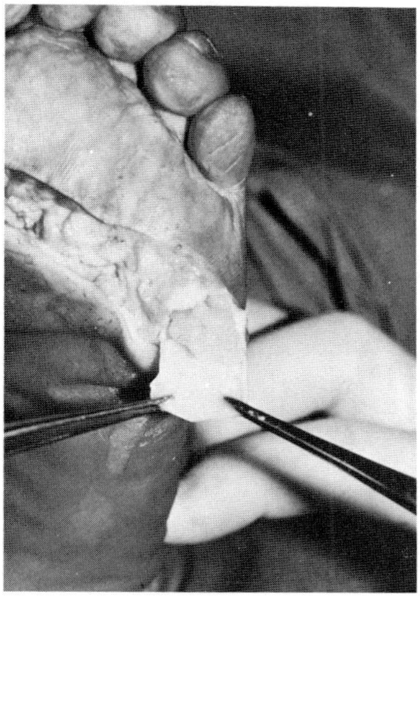

g

After forefoot-arthroplasties the function is of special interest because of long during deformity with contracture of the toes and muscular imbalance. The range of motion is measured by dorsal extension and plantar flexion separately for the hallux and the phalanges. The figure correlating the range of motion versus approach and versus resection shows that two thirds of the group with plantar approach and metatarsal head resection show good motion. The plantar flexion after dorsal approach and additional base resection is in most cases impossible. The relation is shown for phalanges II–V versus resection and for the hallux versus approach (fig. 2, 3). Difficulties during walking can be equalized by shoes. Walking without shoes the results are much better after plantar resection of the metatarsal heads (fig. 4). At the follow-up study, only 5 of 21 patients with plantar approach and 4 of 16 cases with resection of the metatarsal heads needed orthopedic shoes, whereas 19 of 25 cases and 20 of 30 patients of the other group required orthopedic shoes (table V). Because of the additional removal of the heads of the proximal phalanges in cases with claw toes in combination with better realignment of the flexor tendons by the plantar approach we could reduce the number of luxations of the toes at the level of MTP joints (table VI).

Comparing the overall results of patients' and doctors' opinions we can summarize a good result in terms of pain, ability to walk and cosmetic aspects in 80% after plantar approach and 50–60% after dorsal resection (fig. 5, table VII).

Discussion

Resection arthroplasty of the forefoot is one of the most successful operations for rheumatoid patients. Different procedures were established after the first description of Hoffmann in 1911. Pain during walking even after short distances presents the indication in cases where we find destruction and luxations of the metatarsophalangeal joints.

The comparative study of the different procedures of forefoot arthroplasties shows obviously better results for the plantar approach with the resection of the metatarsal heads (fig. 6, 7). The elliptic plantar excision of the sole with resection of the bursae is responsible for a better correction of the phalanges and better relief from pain. The possible realignment of the flexor tendons provides for a better function of the toes. Most of the described procedures do not mention the importance of an additional treatment of the claw toes. We think that the regular resection of the heads of the phalanges helps to prevent a recurrent subluxation of the metatarsophalangeal joint and enforces better function during walking barefoot. It is nearly impossible to correct claw toes operatively in combination with the Clayton-Vainio procedure. Accordingly, with remaining claw toes it is necessary to wear orthopedic shoes. Two thirds of patients after the Clayton-Vainio procedure need orthopedic shoes whereas three quarters with facultative resection of the head of the proximal phalanges use ready-made shoes.

To prevent recurrence of hallux valgus deformity, it is important to pay attention to the metatarsal index described by Lelièvre [1961] and Viladot [1970]. An additional dynamic correction of the great toe can be achieved by refixating the tendon of the m. abductor hallucis dorsally and distally and releasing the lateral sesamoid bone. The arthroplasty of the great toe can be completed by an additional interposition of a capsular flap. In rare cases of a metatarsus I varus deformity it may be necessary to combine the procedure with an osteotomy of the base of the metatarsal I bone [Susman and Clayton, 1983]. Whilst Gschwend et al. [1977] reported as many good results as bad results by plantar approach we correlated better results in terms of pain, function and rehabilitation to the plantar approach especially by isolated resections of the metatarsal heads in combination with a resection of the heads of the proximal phalanges in cases of claw toes. Finally it should be mentioned that a routine regime of postoperative care is important.

Summary

To correct rheumatoid forefoot deformities, several operative procedures by differing approaches are described in the literature. Most of the reported results do not evaluate the influence of the operation on the foot overall. From 1973 to 1983, 97 resection arthroplasties were performed in rheumatoid patients, at the Staatliche Orthopädische Klinik, Munich. The follow-up study of 46 feet shows good results in terms of pain, and ability to walk in 78%. An investigation comparing 25 operations by a dorsal approach and 21 by a plantar approach shows better results for the plantar procedures in terms of pain relief, range of motion, ability to walk and the need for orthopedic shoes. By additional resection of the heads of the proximal phalanges in cases of clawtoe, luxation of the toes was reduced remarkably.

References

Clayton, M.L.: Surgery of the forefoot in rheumatoid arthritis. Clin. Orthop. *16:* 136 (1960).

Fowler, A.W.: A method of forefoot reconstruction. J. Bone Jt Surg. *41B:* 507 (1959).

Gschwend, N.; Barbier, M.; Dybowski, W.R.: Die Vorfusskorrektur. Arch. orthop. Unfallchir. *88:* 75 (1977).

Hoffmann, P.: An operation for severe grades of contracted or clawed toes. Am. J. orthop. Surg. *9:* 441 (1911).

Kates, A.; Kessel, L.; Kay, A.: Arthroplasty of the forefoot. J. Bone Jt Surg. *49B:* 552 (1967).

Lelièvre, J.: Pathologie du pied (Masson, Paris 1952).

Lipscomb, P.R.; Benson, G.M.; Sones, D.A.: Resection of proximal phalanges and metatarsal condyles for deformities of the forefoot due to rheumatoid arthritis. Clin. Orthop. *82:* 24 (1972).

Susman, M.H.; Clayton, M.L.: Surgery of the rheumatoid foot. Am. Acad. Med. *12:* 225-232 (1983).

Tillmann, K.: Operative Behandlung der Polyarthritis - Vorfusskorrektur. Orthopäde *2:* 99 (1973).

Tillmann, K.: Der rheumatische Fuss und seine Behandlung; 1st ed. (Enke, Stuttgart 1977).

Vainio, K.: The rheumatoid foot. A clinical study with pathological and roentgenological comments. Annls Chir. Gynaec. Fenn. *45:* suppl. 1 (1956).

Viladot, A.: Metatarsalgia due to biomechanical alterations of the forefoot. Clin. Orthop. *82:* 24 (1973).

PD Dr. F.-W. Hagena, Rheuma-Einheit der Ludwig-Maximilian-Universität, Staatliche Orthopädische Klinik, Harlachingerstrasse 51, D-8000 München 90 (FRG)

Rheumatology, vol. 11, pp. 173–178 (Karger, Basel 1987)

Resection Arthroplasty versus Arthrodesis of the First Metatarsophalangeal Joint for Hallux Valgus in Rheumatoid Arthritis

Pauli Raunio, Mauri Lehtimäki, Matti Eerola, Martti Hämäläinen, Tapio Pulkki

Rheumatism Foundation Hospital, Heinola, Finland

Introduction

As arthrodesis of the first metatarsophalangeal joint (MTP I) has in general been condemned in the treatment of the rheumatoid hallux valgus (HV), we decided to perform a retrospective comparative study of patients who were operated in years 1981–82 with either *resection arthroplasty* or *arthrodesis* of the MTP I for HV in order to see, whether arthrodesis is justified or not.

Material and Methods

Table I shows our material. 27 patients in both resection and arthrodesis groups. Males accounted for only one sixth in the resection group and one third in the arthrodesis group. There were 35 MTP I joints in resections and 30 MTP I joints in arthrodeses operated upon. Mean age was about the same (53–54 years) in both, but follow-up time was a year longer in the resection group.

Results

In table II the functional and anatomical results are shown *as the doctor has seen and evaluated them.* One can see that at least three quarters came off fairly well in the light of these figures. The arthrodesis group seems to succeed a bit better but not to a significant extent. Table

Table I. Resection arthroplasty vs arthrodesis for hallux valgus

Material	Resections	Arthrodeses
Patients	27	27
Males: females	4:23	7:20
MTPI joints operated upon	35	30
of which unilateral	19	24
of which bilateral	16	6
Mean age, years	53 ± 9	54 ± 10
Mean follow-up time, months	44 ± 30	31 ± 8

Table II. Arthroplasty vs arthrodesis

Results: doctor's evaluation	Resections (n = 35)			Arthrodeses (n = 30)		
	n	%		n	%	
Functional						
Excellent or good	16	46	} 80	15	50	} 93
Fair	12	34		13	43	
Poor	7	20		2	7	n.s.
Anatomical						
Excellent or good	14	40	} 77	16	53	} 83
Fair	13	37		9	30	
Poor	8	23		5	17	n.s.

Table III. Arthroplasty vs arthrodesis

Results: patient's evaluation	Resections (n = 35)		Arthrodeses (n = 30)	
	n	%	n	%
Much better–better	28	80	23	77
Unchanged	4	11	4	13
Worse	3	9	3	10

Table IV. Arthroplasty vs arthrodesis

	Resections (n = 35), %	Arthrodeses (n = 30), %
Causes of satisfaction		
Pain gone or reduced	60	43
Bunion disappeared	43	43
Position of great toe better	34	50 n.s.
Able to wear ordinary shoes	37	36
Causes of dissatisfaction		
Persistent pain in MTPI	20	6
Persistent bunion	9	6
Deformity recurred	43	10 n.s.
Great toe in hyperextension	*17*	*27*
Poor movement in MTPI	*29*	*23*
Swelling or other discomfort	–	13

Table V. Arthroplasty vs arthrodesis. The influence of metatarsus primus varus on hallux valgus and respective operative corrections of hallux valgus

	Group[a]	MTI/II angle, °	Preop. HV angle, °	Extent of correction, °	Postop. HV angle,°	Target angle, °	Shortage of correct., °	Number of fact
Resection patients	I	*5*	*22*	6	16	15	*1*	10
	II	*8*	*30*	7	23	18	5	12
	III	*10*	*36*	11	25	20	5	13
	Total	8	31	10	21	18	3	35
Arthrodesis patients		8	31	15	16	18	–	30

[a] Group I: 5 ± 2.1°; II: 8 ± 0°; III: 10 ± 2°.

III shows how *the patient has estimated* the outcome of the operations. The figures are very close to those of the doctor's evaluation, and again no significant difference is evident between groups.

The analysis of the *reasons for satisfaction and dissatisfaction* is shown in table IV. Causes of satisfaction are much the same in both groups but there are a couple of reasons for dissatisfaction which are

a

b

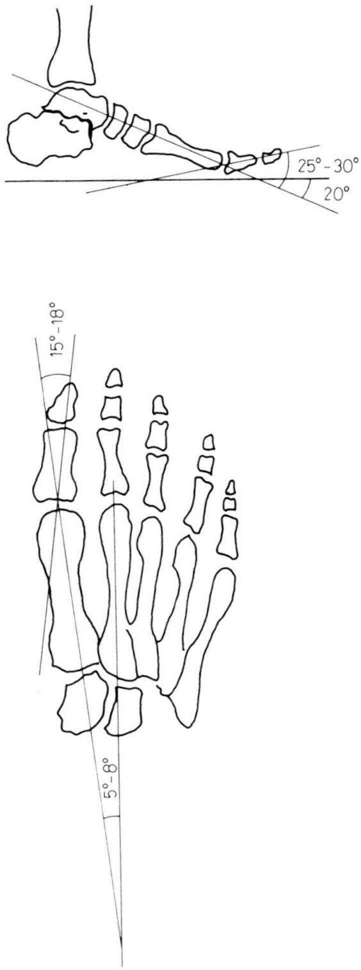

Fig. 1. a Extension position, and TSJ *b* valgus position recommended by the authors for arthrodesis of the first metatarsophalangeal joint.

interesting. In the resection group there were too many people dissatisfied with recurring HV or other deformity, e.g. hyperextension. In this point the difference between groups is, if not significant, yet indicative, i.e. the risk of chance is about 10%. Note also that poor movement causes dissatisfaction less frequently in fusion than in the resection group. Paradoxical, isn't it?

Table V shows *how the increasing angle of the first and second metatarsals influences the HV angle.* The resection material was divided into three classes according to MT I/II angle as follows: group I: 5° ± 2°; II: 8° ± 0°, III: 10° ± 2°. The arthrodesis group appears as one group with an approximate MT I/II angle of 8 ± 3°.

The correlation between MT I/II angle and HV angle is clear. Table V shows also the target HV angle and the correction achieved by the operation in each above group. If HV and MT I/II angles are small the correction is nearly complete, whereas a greater deformity seems to leave greater shortage of correction. Probably the correction even in these cases has originally been adequate but deteriorated in the course of time, at least partly due to excess of MT I/II angle. According to our experience osteotomy of the first metatarsal should be considered if the MT I/II angle is greater than 10°.

Scrutiny of the causes of dissatisfaction revealed that all patients who had the great toe base fused in more than 35° or less than 20° of extension were displeased with the outcome. These experiences have resulted in the recommendation to position the great toe in 25° of extension for men and in 30° for women. This means 10–5° of extension from the floor plane. In these two figures we have collected the *essential information achieved by this study:* (fig. 1a) the great toe should be positioned in 25–30° of extension; (fig. 1b) the advisable HV angle is the angle between the first and second metatarsals increased by 10°.

Even if the resection and arthrodesis groups do not significantly differ from each other, we can conclude that almost all failures in the arthrodesis group could have been avoided by proper technique. In the resection method the main causes of dissatisfaction are not so clear and not so easy to eliminate. However, arthrodesis of the MTP I joint has proven to be a good alternative in the treatment of MTP I and rheumatoid arthritis. In certain cases it is preferable to any other method.

Summary

Thirty-five resection arthroplasties of the first metatarsophalangeal (MTP I) joint for rheumatoid hallux valgus were compared with thirty MTP I arthrodeses. Functional and anatomical assessments of the results, performed by the doctor as well as by the patient, did not reveal significant superiority to either of the series. They did reveal, however, that the failures of the arthrodeses almost constantly resulted from incorrect positioning of the fusion. These can be avoided by proper technique. More than 30° of extension was mostly felt troublesome by the patient, and the same was true if the angle was less than 25°. In the resection method, on the contrary, the failures cannot readily be avoided by better technique. The preoperative degree of hallux valgus depends largely on the degree of metatarsus primus varus (the angle of the first and second metatarsals), and this fact is to be borne in mind when positioning the hallux valgus angulation at the operation. We recommend that this angulation be calculated as follows: The angle between the first and second metatarsals increased by 10° results in recommendable valgus angle for MTP I correction, both in resection arthroplasty and in arthrodesis. Osteotomy of the first metatarsal is worth consideration if the MTP I–II angle is greater than 6–7°. If these rules are kept the overall results of arthrodesis are certainly better than those of resection. In the latter method hallux valgus often recurs or other deformities, like hyperextension or varus deviation, occur.

Pauli Raunio, MD, Rheumatism Foundation Hospital, Rautsalo C 9,
SF-18100 Heinola 10 (Finland)

Rheumatology, vol. 11, pp. 179–187 (Karger, Basel 1987)

The Complex Foot

Synovectomy of the Ankle and Subtalar Joints. Total Replacement Arthroplasty of the Ankle Joint

Jan A. Pahle, Jens C. Teigland

Oslo Sanitetsforening Rheumatism Hospital, Oslo, Norway

Introduction

Whereas arthritis of the talocrural joint according to Vainio [9] occurs in only 9% of patients with rheumatoid arthritis, the subtalar joints and the joints constituting Chopart's joint are affected in 62–70% in different materials. Our own experience concurs with that of Jakubowski [4, 5] who found that about 50% of patients with rheumatoid arthritis have affection of the talocrural and subtalar joints, very often simultaneously, in other words almost as frequently as affection of the wrist. The affection of the ankle and hindfoot have, however, been given very low priority in cases of multiple affections. Destructions in these joints cause severe invalidity and every effort should be given to prevent these destructions. It is interesting that in juvenile rheumatoid arthritis of pauciarticular type, the ankle joint is affected in combination with the ipsilateral knee joint in about 60%. In juvenile cases growth disturbances in the actual epiphyseal areas may have more significance than the destructive process itself.

Synovitis of the talocrural joint gives rise to swelling around one or both malleoli, and as a rule also anteriorly. Very often a simultaneous tenosynovitis is present, which is not always easy to diagnose because of a tendency to edema in the ankle region.

Because of the distension of the joint capsule and affection of the ligaments, instability is often seen whereby talus will tilt in the ankle mortice or is movable forwards as in an anterior drawer symptom of the knee. Later on when the destructions are pronounced, restricted motion is a usual finding. The patients have only rarely pain at rest in the talocrural joint. The pain on weight bearing is also much less pronounced than one should expect from the radiological findings.

Of 14,200 operations performed on rheumatoid patients in the years 1968 through 1984 in Oslo Sanitetsforening Rheumatism Hospital, synovectomy of the talocrural and tarsal joints amount to a total number of 158 cases – a rather modest share of the total number of synovectomies, probably too modest. In the same period 66 total replacement arthroplasties of the talocrural joint have been performed.

Material and Methods

Synovectomy

With refined technique [5, 6, 8, 10] synovectomy of the talocrural and subtarsal joints is giving no less satisfactory results than in other locations of the disease. The results after up to 17 years follow-up seem highly convincing. Between 1968 and 1976 synovectomy was performed in altogether 63 ankle joints who all had swelling and most of them pain on weight bearing (table I). Radiologically most of these ankle joints were grade II according to the Larsen/Dale/Eek standardization. Age at the time of operation ranged between 7 and 66 years, average 42 years.

The synovial membranes of the actual joints may be reached through 3 incisions, one longitudinal anterior and 2 curved incisions behind the lateral and medial malleolus, respectively, sometimes with partial discission of ligaments. Tenosynovectomy on the 7 most important tendons is done if necessary [2]. Partial rupture of the tendons have been observed several times. Through the anterior approach both malleoli and the trochlea tali are easily reached. The subtalar joints may be reached through one of the curved posterior incisions. The dilatation of the joint capsule facilitates the access to the joint. The talofibular and posterior talotibial ligaments as well as the posterior part of the deltoid ligament must sometimes be partially divided, but usually vital ligaments are left intact. Simple suture of the severed ligaments is enough. Postoperative immobilization is very seldom necessary, active excercises should be started immediately, and partial weight bearing in a supporting boot permitted after 3 weeks.

Table I. Arthritis of talocrural and tarsal joints (n = 63)

Swelling	63
Pain on weight bearing	55
X-Ray: Grade I	9
Grade II	40
Grade III	14

Table II. Synovectomy of talocrural and tarsal joints. Results after 5.7 years (n = 63)

	Preoperative	Postoperative
Pain on weight bearing	55	17
Swelling	63	22
Instability	38	17
Range of movement, mean (46 increased)	15°	32°

Results

In 21 of 38 patients where a preoperative instability was diagnosed, an appreciable improvement of stability was found on postoperative examination (table II). Postoperative bowstringing of the tendons may be avoided by a meticulous closure of the fibrous tendon sheath. No deleterious effect of ankle synovectomy in children has been observed. It is possible that synovectomy has been beneficial to the growth disturbances which is a regular finding in juvenile rheumatoid arthritis. This is, however, more obvious in other joints.

At the follow-up 46 of 63 ankles were found to be free of pain on weight bearing, 10 cases had a tolerable pain, and in 7 cases the pain was severe and led to arthrodesis in 5 and arthroplasty in 2 cases. The improved stability was marked [7], but on the other hand there was a reduced range of motion in 17 ankles. In 46 ankle joints, which all were pain-free, the range of motion had increased 25° on average.

During the same 9 years from 1968 to 1976 arthrodesis of the ankle joint was performed in 21 cases as the first operation, a ratio synovectomy versus arthrodesis of 3:1. After 1976 arthrodesis of the talocrural joint has not been performed in our hospital.

It is more difficult to assess the value of synovectomy of the subtalar and Chopart's joints, although some patients are doing very well 14 years postoperatively. The invalidity caused by a triple arthrodesis is almost negligible [1] and this operation has been one of the most appreciated by the patients and has been performed in 221 feet. It is interesting to note that whereas rather small erosions in the subtalar joints lead to pain upon weight bearing at an early stage of the disease, the patients with rather advanced radiological destructions in the ankle mortice are able to walk around without complaining of much pain. For this reason many patients with affection of the ankle joint come very late for synovectomy.

Arthroplasty

Arthroplasty of the ankle joint is very seldom indicated in monoarticular disease, as for example post-traumatic osteoarthritis. The invalidity caused by an arthrodesed ankle joint in correct position is very small, and well accepted, especially if the foot is equipped with a shoe with a shock-absorbing heel.

If the neighbouring joints are affected, however, a stiff ankle joint is not very well tolerated, and especially not if the patient has an ipsilateral stiff knee. In rheumatoid arthritis where multiple joint affections are very likely to occur, one should always be reluctant to fuse a joint.

Arthroplasty of the ankle joint has therefore been the treatment of choice in such cases. The results of prophylactic synovectomy of the ankle joint, however, are encouraging [7, 8] and may well have contributed to preservation of many ankle joints.

From 1975 through 1984 66 arthroplasties in the ankle joint were performed (table III), all with a modified Thompson prosthesis. The great majority of the patients suffered from rheumatoid arthritis or juvenile arthritis. There were also 2 haemophiliacs during these years, with satisfactory long-term results (table IV).

34 of the patients were on steroids. The youngest patient was 15 years of age. Average age at the time of operation was 45 years. Two of the patients had earlier had a synovectomy of the ankle and were now reoperated because of persistent pain during weight bearing. The others had not been operated earlier in the ankle joint. In one case the main indication was varus deformity. In 4 cases ankylosis was the indication (table V).

The observation time of these patients is on an average 5 years. The degree of radiological destruction was considerable, usually grade IV–V in our scale. Corresponding to the degree of destruction of the ankle mortice almost all had moderate to considerable pain on weight bearing. There was no instability on clinical examination preoperatively, no drawer symptom, but 7 had a sensation of instability when walking. 4 had ankylotic ankle joints and the remainder had a motion preoperatively reduced to an average of $-1°$ dorsiflexion and $19°$ plantarflexion.

Table III. TRP ankle prosthesis (n = 66)

Female 52	Male 14
Age, mean 45 years (15–68)	
On steroids 34 (51%)	

Table IV. TRP ankle prosthesis (1975–1984)

Arthritis rheumatoides	43
Arthritis juvenilis	18
Mb. Bechterew	1
Osteoarthritis	2
Haemophilia	2
Total number	66

Table V. TRP ankle prosthesis. Main indication for operation (n = 66)

Pain	61
Varus deformities	1
Ankylosis	4

Technique

A modified version of the Thompson-Parkridge-Richards ankle prosthesis has been used in all 66 cases. Through a longitudinal anterior incision in the midline, the transverse and cruciate ligaments are divided. The extensor hallucis longus and the tibialis anterior tendons are pulled medially, and the neurovascular bundle laterally. The fibrous capsule is opened through a longitudinal incision. It is often very thin, covered with fatty tissue. It is important to preserve as much as possible of the capsule and the extra-articular fat in order to ensure good soft-tissue covering of the prosthesis. In preparing the bed for the prosthesis the ankle spacer will secure correct alignment and size of the prosthesis. It is important to restrict the osteotomy as much as possible towards the medial malleolus in order to avoid fracture at the base of the malleolus. Using the talus template as a guide, a hole is drilled into the talus for the peg of the talus component. A sagittal slot is reamed by means of an air drill with a small ball reamer, and in order to ensure recession of the edge of the talus prosthesis, a shallow groove is reamed on the joint surface of the trochlea tali for the edge of the prosthesis. To ensure correct alignment of the tibial section, a guiding handle for the trial prosthesis as well as for the permanent prosthesis of the tibial part has been developed. This handle is equipped with a guiding pin which should point towards patella parallel to tibia both from a frontal and side view. The talus and tibial trial prostheses are tested assembled in situ several times. Every endeavour should be made to ensure optimal adaptation of the two halves of the prosthesis against bone, to obtain a stable position during motion even before cementation. The parts of talus which project medially and laterally to the talus prosthesis often have to be resected to prevent collision with the flanges of the tibial prosthesis. The permanent talus prosthesis is cemented first. In the setting phase of the cement, correct positioning of the prosthesis is ensured by pressing the talus against the tibia trial prosthesis. Thereafter the tibial section is cemented. The guiding handle should be used in both procedures to ensure the correct position in all three planes. Without this guiding handle there is a great tendency to tilt the tibia prosthesis in a distal direction dorsally.

The joint is swilled thoroughly with saline solution and inspected for any impinging particles of bone or cement. The movement between the two surfaces should be tested. It should be a sliding movement, not a hinge movement. The range of motion before closure of the soft tissues is about 40° totally. The fibrous capsule with the periarticular fat is closed in layers. The crural fascia with its ligamentous reinforcements is closed meticulously superficial to the tendons to prevent bowstringing. Immobilization in a plaster cast has not been necessary. Active dorsal and plantar motions are started on the first postoperative day, and partial weight bearing will usually be permitted after 2 weeks.

If the subtalar joints are affected, indicating a triple arthrodesis, this should be done prior to a total replacement arthroplasty of the ankle joint.

Results

The follow-up has been up to 9.5 years, on average 5 years. Postoperatively almost all patients are free of pain (table VI). The pain has been graded according to a 0–3 scale (ARO) which shows a rather remarkable reduction postoperatively [3]. The stability is also quite good, and more than half of the patients are able to walk tiptoe on the operated foot. In one case it was not possible to correct completely the varus deformity because of the rather severe destructions of talus. 16 of the patients have a feeling of some stiffness, but all have a satisfactory range of motion with an average dorsiflexion postoperatively of 6° and a plantar flexion of 20° (table VII). The plantar flexion is seemingly

Table VI. TRP ankle prosthesis. Pain (ARO: 0 = none, 1 = slight, 2 = moderate, 3 = severe)

Preoperative: Mean 2.2	Postoperative: Mean 0.3

Table VII. TRP ankle prosthesis. Range of motion

	Preoperative	Postoperative
Dorsal motion	− 1° (−30 to 30)	+ 6° (−7 to 15)
Plantar motion	+19° (0–45)	+20° (5–45)

Table VIII. TRP ankle prosthesis. Early complications

Infections	
Superficial	2
Deep	0
Delayed wound healing	18
Skin grafted	2
Canalis tarsi syndrome	1

small, but sufficient for the gait. The pain-free ankle has given the patients a larger radius of action, and has also in some cases seemingly improved the function of the knee.

Complications

Among the early complications (table VIII) delayed wound healing has been somewhat bothersome. In 2 cases skin grafting was necessary. It does not seem to matter very much how the incisions are made, but the skin should be handled with utmost care like in hand surgery. In one case the patient developed a tarsal tunnel syndrome which necessitated decompression. Later on loosening of the prosthetic parts occurred in 3 cases (table IX).

In one case talus collapsed almost completely and the prosthetic parts had to be removed. An arthrodesis was attempted, but the healing was delayed very much, and was not quite solid when the patient died recently of a heart failure. In 2 other cases the tibial component was found to be loose. In one case refixation was successful. In the other the prosthesis was removed completely and a successful arthrodesis was achieved by means of a 3-flanged hip nail driven up from the plantar side of calcaneus into tibia.

New bone formation between talus and the medial malleolus have necessitated a small revision in 3 cases. We have had no cases of late infections. In the patient's own assessment the results are satisfactory (table X) in more than 80% of the cases [3].

Table IX. TRP ankle prosthesis. Late complications

Loosening:	Tibia	2
	Talus	1
Collapse of talus:		1
New bone formation talus/med. malleolus:		3

Table X. TRP ankle prosthesis. Patient's opinion

	Number	Percent
Good	55	83
Fair	10	15.5
Bad	1	1.5

Discussion

The results of synovectomy of the talocrural and subtalar joints are encouraging, indicating a prophylactic value. Triple arthrodesis is a beneficial procedure. When indicated it should be done prior to talocrural arthroplasty. Talocrural arthrodesis should be avoided in patients suffering from rheumatoid arthritis. The results after 5 years observation time after arthroplasty of the talocrural joint in rheumatoid patients are satisfactory. It is felt that the side flanges of the tibial prosthesis may have played an important role in assuring side stability.

The number of registered loosenings in these patients where osteoporosis is so prevalent is within acceptable limits, probably because the demands on the prosthesis are less in rheumatoid patients than in monoarticular osteoarthritis (less body weight, less muscle power, less action).

Summary

The technique of synovectomy of the ankle and subtalar joint is described. Synovectomy was performed in 63 ankles with a follow-up time up to 7 years. A significant reduction of pain and instability has been noted. 46 ankle joints were all pain-free with an increased range of motion. In 7 cases an arthrodesis (5) or arthroplasty (2) had to be performed later on because of persistent pain.

Since 1975, 66 arthroplasties in the ankle joint have been performed. The indications, technique and results are described. Observation time, 5 years. A good and lasting result regarding pain and stability has been achieved with an average dorsiflexion of 6° and plantarflexion of 20°. Delayed wound healing and one case of nerve impingement were the early complications. The tibial component became loose in 2 cases, and in one case talus collapsed completely. Talocrural arthrodesis should be avoided in patients suffering from rheumatoid arthritis. The number of registered loosenings is within acceptable limits. When indicated, a triple arthrodesis should be done prior to arthroplasty of the talocrural joint.

References

1 Clayton, M.L.: Situation of the foot regarding early synovectomy in RA. Symp. on Early Synovectomy in Rheumatoid Arthritis, Amsterdam 1967.
2 Dybowski, W.R.: Surgical treatment of rheumatoid tenosynovitis at the feet. Chir. Narzadow Ruchu Ortop. Pol. *30:* 563 (1965).
3 Engelbrecht, E.: Sprunggelenksendoprothese Modell 'St. Georg'. Z. Orthop. *113:* 546 (1975).
4 Jakubowski, S.: Discussion. Symp. on Early Synovectomy in Rheumatoid Arthritis, Amsterdam 1967.
5 Jakubowski, S.: Synovektomie des oberen Sprunggelenks. Orthopäde *2:* 79 (1973).
6 Meier, G.; Bontemps, G.; Tillmann, K.: Synovektomie des oberen Sprunggelenkes bei rheumatischer Arthritis. Ortop. Praxis *11:* 874 (1975).
7 Tillmann, K.: The rheumatoid foot (Thieme, Stuttgart 1979).
8 Vahvanen, V.S.: Synovectomy of the talocrural joint in rheumatoid arthritis. Annls Chir. Gynaec. Fenn. *57:* 576 (1968).
9 Vainio, K.: The rheumatoid foot. Annls Chir. Gynaec. Fenn. suppl. 1, p. 45 (1956).
10 Wilkinson, M.C.; Lowry, J.H.: Synovectomy for rheumatoid arthritis. J. Bone Jt Surg. *47B:* 482 (1965).

Prof. Jan A. Pahle, MD, Oslo Sanitetsforening Rheumatism Hospital,
Akersbakken 27, N-0172 Oslo 1 (Norway)

Subject Index